Fulton, F. L. The medical language: divide and conquer.
Harrington Read Pubishing Company. Ruxton-Riderwood: Maryland, 2010.

ISBN#: 978-0-9824128-0-0

Production Manager: Emily Read
Senior Editor: R. Meehe
Editorial Assistant: L. Dudley
Managing Editor: Nell Buberry
Lead Designer: E. F. Kemp

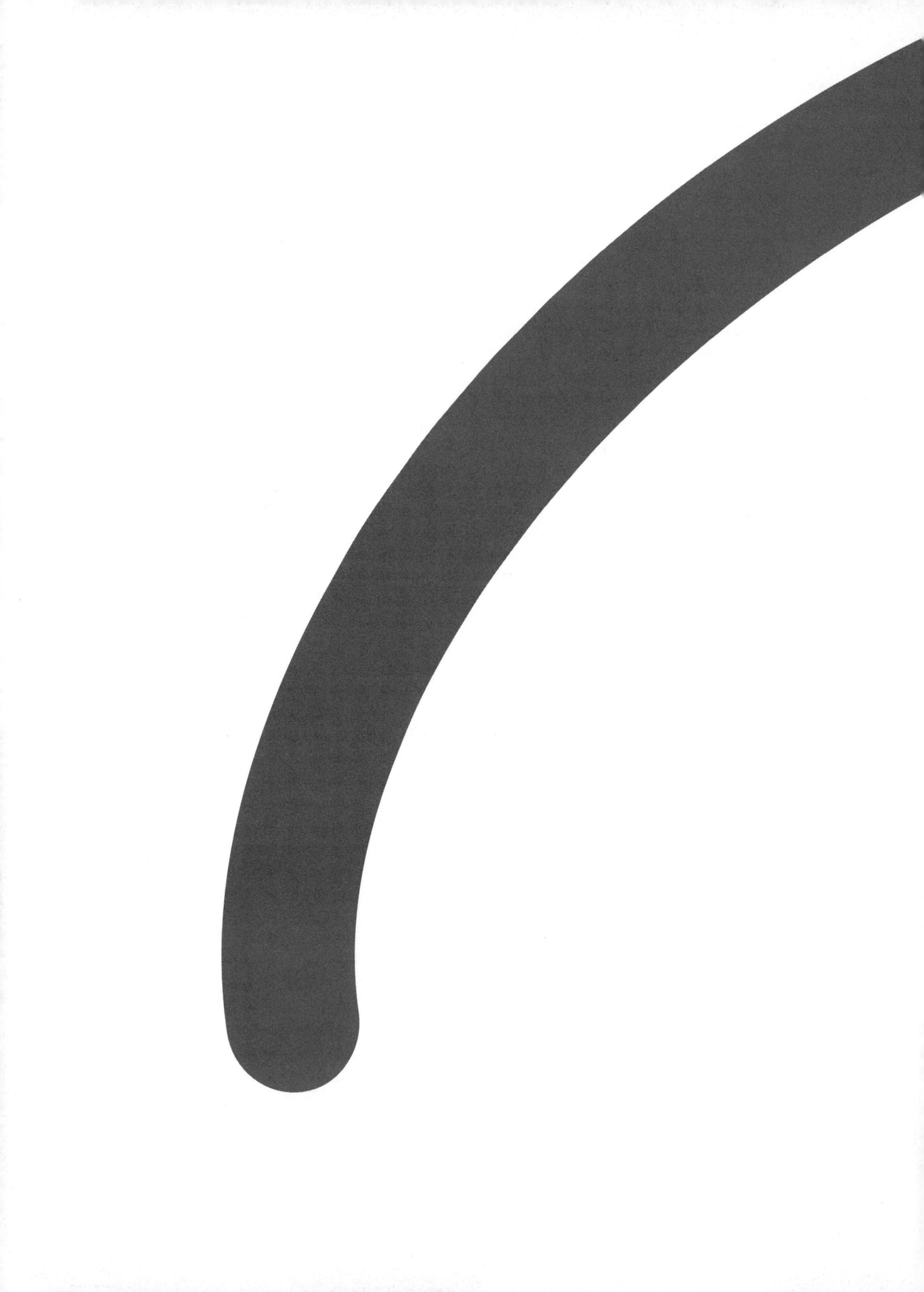

The Medical Language:
Divide and Conquer

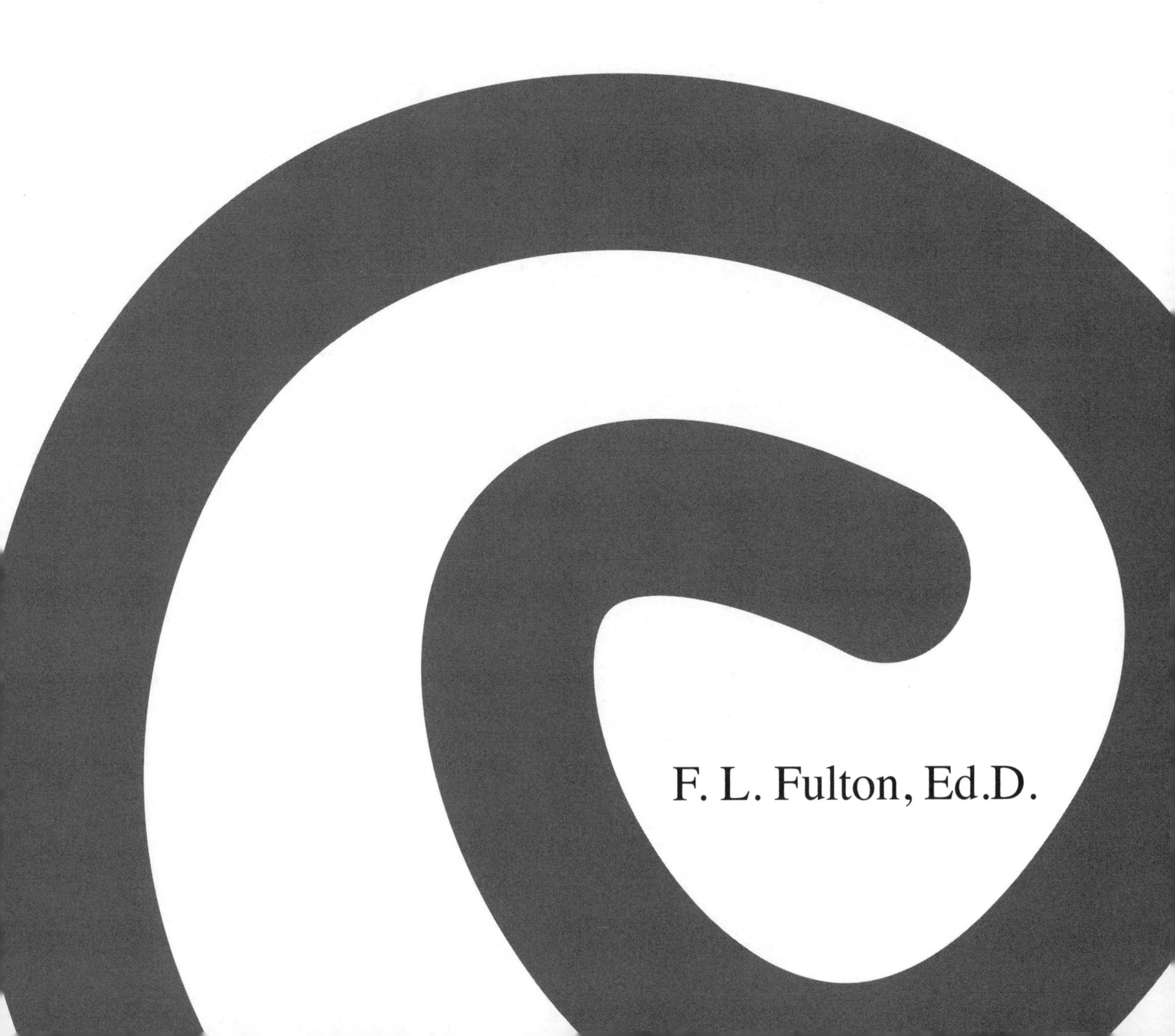

F. L. Fulton, Ed.D.

The Medical Language:
Divide and Conquer

F. L. Fulton, M.S., C.A.S., C.A.S.E., Ed.D.

ISBN#: 978-0-9824128-0-0

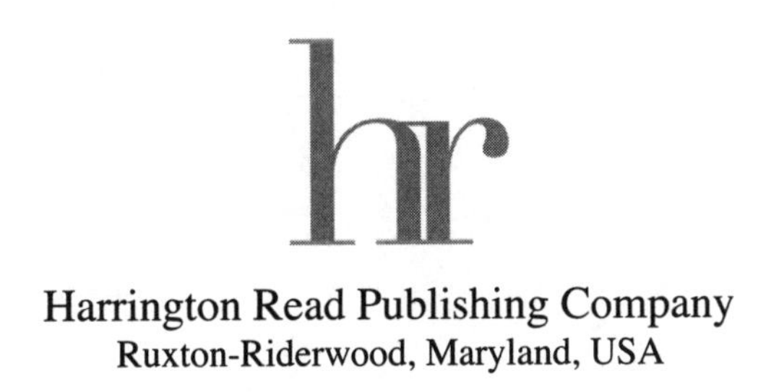

Harrington Read Publishing Company
Ruxton-Riderwood, Maryland, USA

Preface

Target Audience. This is a no-frills and bottom line presentation of the essential medical terms to know. It offers a lean but thorough presentation of the topic at a most reasonable price for students on a tight budget. Moreover, this text transcends the status quo. With nearly twenty years of teaching college level Medical Terminology, the author designed the practice exercises to be to be creative, non-intimidating, fun, laid back, and/ or memorable to enhance the ease of medical term application. Specifically, this text is designed for a wide variety of differently learning abled students. Generally; the audience is anyone interested in allied health education, such as medical administration assistants, medical records specialists, and medical receptionists. Unit coordinators, physical therapists, and surgical technologists will also be an appropriate audience. Laboratory technologists, radiology technologists, and veterinary assistants. Acupuncturists, massage therapists, occupational therapists, physician assistants and acupressurists. Certified nursing assistants, home health aides, hospice helpers, and dialysis technicians. Surgical technicians, L.P.N./L.V.N.s, R.N.s, and E.N.D. technicians. Chiropractic assistants, E.E.G. technicians, and insurance adjusters. Paralegal assistants, attorneys, legal administrative assistants, and law students. Pharmaceutical aides and health care employees. Sports medicine specialists and educators. Phlebotomy technicians, paramedics, and medical lab assistants. Increasingly, this text appeals to anyone interested in familiarizing themselves with the language of medicine.

Text Objective

To support student's success and joy in learning tools to tackle new medical terms, this textbook is designed for student friendly assistance in learning medical terminology as an independent study or a group classroom course. By dividing medical terms down into smaller components, new students learn to succeed. Moreover, a refreshing approach to student success will be introduced and exercised. While most textbooks are geared to only visual and auditory learning, this textbook will offer more ways for terms to be approached with common sense and logical sequence that promotes a thorough understanding and foundation upon which to build new words.

As there are abundant online resources, this book is designed to provide a very reasonably priced and student friendly basic reference that employs multiple dimensions of learning. It is also a diving board foundation from which to leap toward 'going green' with the myriad of free, high quality and creative online learning opportunities.

Instead of the same old limited approach of only memorizing new medical terms, this text comprehensively addresses some practices utilizing a broad range of learning dimensions. For example: language learners will particularly enjoy writing or speaking practices. Logical learners will shine when order and number manipulation are employed. Spatial learners will have practice in creative art to best learn. Body learners will have the opportunity to assimilate knowledge via body movement and action. Musical learners may absorb terms better when presented in rhythm or pitch patterns. As people learners attend to mood and motives behind medical terms, these issues will be addressed. Self learners will have the chance to apply terms to their real life situations. Nature learners characteristically practice new words in the natural world. Moreover, this textbook assumes no prior knowledge of medical terms. Embracing a diverse student population, this textbook seeks to focus on individual progress from wherever the student's learning baseline is. Instead of just a traditional mode of a boring rote memorization, student success will be enhanced by approaching new terms with an adventurous spirit in exercises of practical application.

Acknowledgements

Thanks to students, I have been inspired to design this text to better meet an ever changing and diverse population. Utilizing a student centered methodology, this text endeavors to facilitate each student's learning style regardless of their previous professional experience or lack thereof.

Sincere gratitude is extended to T. R., H. L. Bryan, M. T. Sidhwani, and M. E. Harrington. E. R. Fulton's tirelesss effort and time is especially greatly appreciated..

F. L. Fulton

TABLE OF CONTENTS

Introduction

Learning Medical Terms

There is more than one way to "skin a cat". Whereas learning styles look at how we learn, intelligence refers to our abilities to solve problems. A Harvard professor, named Howard Gardner, maintains that a singular number produced when measuring intelligence (IQ) is misleading as we actually possess eight intelligences we can utilize anytime we tackle a learning project. Linquistic intelligence refers to an ability to express oneself well in writing and speech. Logical-mathematical intelligence relates to the understanding of cause/effect, abstract thinking, logic, order, number manipulation, and problem solving abilities. Spatial intelligence targets the capabilities of visual re-creation and sense of direction. Bodily-kinesthetic intelligence is the ability to learn via coordinated body control, movement, and action. Musical intelligence focuses on the strengths of pattern recognition, rhythm, and pitch. Interpersonal intelligence attends to the comprehension of other's moods and motive. Intrapersonal intelligence focuses on self understanding. Naturalistic intelligence relates to a unique ability to explain, understand, relate, classify, and separate characteristics in the natural world. Everyone has dominant intelligences as well as less well developed intelligences. By identifying and understanding your dominant intelligences as a student, you will be better armed for maximum benefit from tailored study. As teachers; the more varied intelligences that are exercised in facilitating learning in the classroom, the better the outcome for students.

Visual learners will be best assisted by well-organized interesting supplemental visual material. Power Point presentations, computer C.D.s, D.V.D.s, overhead projections, video camera outputs, podcasts, live video feeds, Internet, posters, maps, films, closed circuit television, slide shows, photographs, and other visual products would be especially helpful learning tools, along with visually appealing handouts. When studying; it is helpful to be alone in a quiet location, to rewrite every medical term five to ten times each, to utilize color to highlight the more challenging medical terms on flashcards, and to review all visual material highlights.

Auditory learners often find it helpful to sit close to the source of classroom information (the teacher, the speaker, etc.) that incorporates multimedia applications using sounds, speech, and /or music. With the instructor's permission, it may assist the student to record each class. The teacher's attention to aural textures while rephrasing highlights of the classroom would be helpful. The volume, pitch, and speed variations of particularly important points would reinforce the material when studying. It may assist auditory learners to recite information with a study-buddy, to create a rhyme or song for more difficult terms, to read aloud flashcards of every new medical term with the definition, and to listen to recordings of the class so that you may hear the words as you study them.

Tactile-kinesthetic learners may benefit most from classroom demonstrations involving movement and hands-on activity. By allowing breaks every twenty minutes during lessons, these students are better able to re-focus on the subject. While studying, it may be helpful for the student to handle a safe, squishy object for grounding, to take frequent three to five minute breaks, and to practice learning games. Some potential exercises/game options may include medical term hangman, bingo, jeopardy, and concentration.

While memorization is a basic necessity to succeed in this course, I hope you will avail yourself to the myriad of chapter exercises that incorporate the use of more of your various intelligences. Whatever your learning styles, play to your strengths!

Pronunciation Before You Start 4-1-1 Assistance

A macron ( ) is added over the vowels with a long vowel sound. For example: a=day, e=be, i=kite, o=no, u=universe. A breve ( ) is provided over the vowels with a short vowel sound. For example: a=alone, e=ever, i=sit, o=ton, u=fun.

PRONUNCIATIONS	WORD EXAMPLES
c (before a, o, u) = k	cavity, colon
c (before e, i) = s	cephalic, cirrhisis
ch = k	cholesterol, cholecytitis
g (before a, o, u) = g	gallstone, gonad
g (before e, i) = j	generic, giant
ph = f	phonetics, pharyngitis
pn = n	pneumonia, pneumothorax
ps = s	psychology
pt = t	ptosis, pterygium
rh = r	rhythm, rhinitis
rrh = r	hemorrhoid, hemorrhage
x = z (when the first letter)	xerosis

Chapter 1

Getting To The Root

Starting medical terminology is like studying the process of making a sandwich or a house. Medical terms, sandwiches, and houses all have building materials. Like a house foundation or the middle of a sandwich, the most important element of a medical term is a root word part.

Although only a medical term can be used in a sentence, a root word part is an essential element of a medical term. The root is like the meat in a sandwich or the foundation for the house. Building a medical term is as easy as "1-2-3."

The bottom line is that all of the root word parts will need to be memorized as they are the foundation for most of the medical terms in this book. Hence, the next page is your visual study guide. Moreover, you will need to know the medical terms you will create at the end of the chapter practice exercises. These medical terms are essential for what you'll need to succeed.

Step 1:

Next you'll see how to build a medical term starting with the root word parts.

Step 2:

In addition to familiarizing yourself with these root word parts, you will need other ingredients in order to build a medical term. Like the sandwich analogy, the root word part is the meat or cheese in your sandwich and the suffix (a word part at the end of a term) is the slice of bread that finishes a sandwich or makes a medical term useable as a word in a sentence. Like a finishing nail when building a house, the suffix holds the root word part structure together to build a whole medical term that may then be appropriately spoken or written.

The following suffixes will need to be learned in order to know some new medical terms. A suffix (usually preceeded by "-" as a symbol of that suffix) needs a root word part added to form a medical term. The "-" is dropped when the root word part is added to form a medical term.

-y	(process or procedure of)
-ology	(process or procedure of, study or science of)
-itis	(inflammation of)
-ectomy	(process or procedure of surgically excising, cutting out, or removing)

Step 3:

It is important to practice putting all of the root word parts together with these suffixes to create as many possible medical terms as possible. You will need to know how to spell all of these medical terms and to define each term properly should you encounter them. For example:

ROOT WORD PARTS

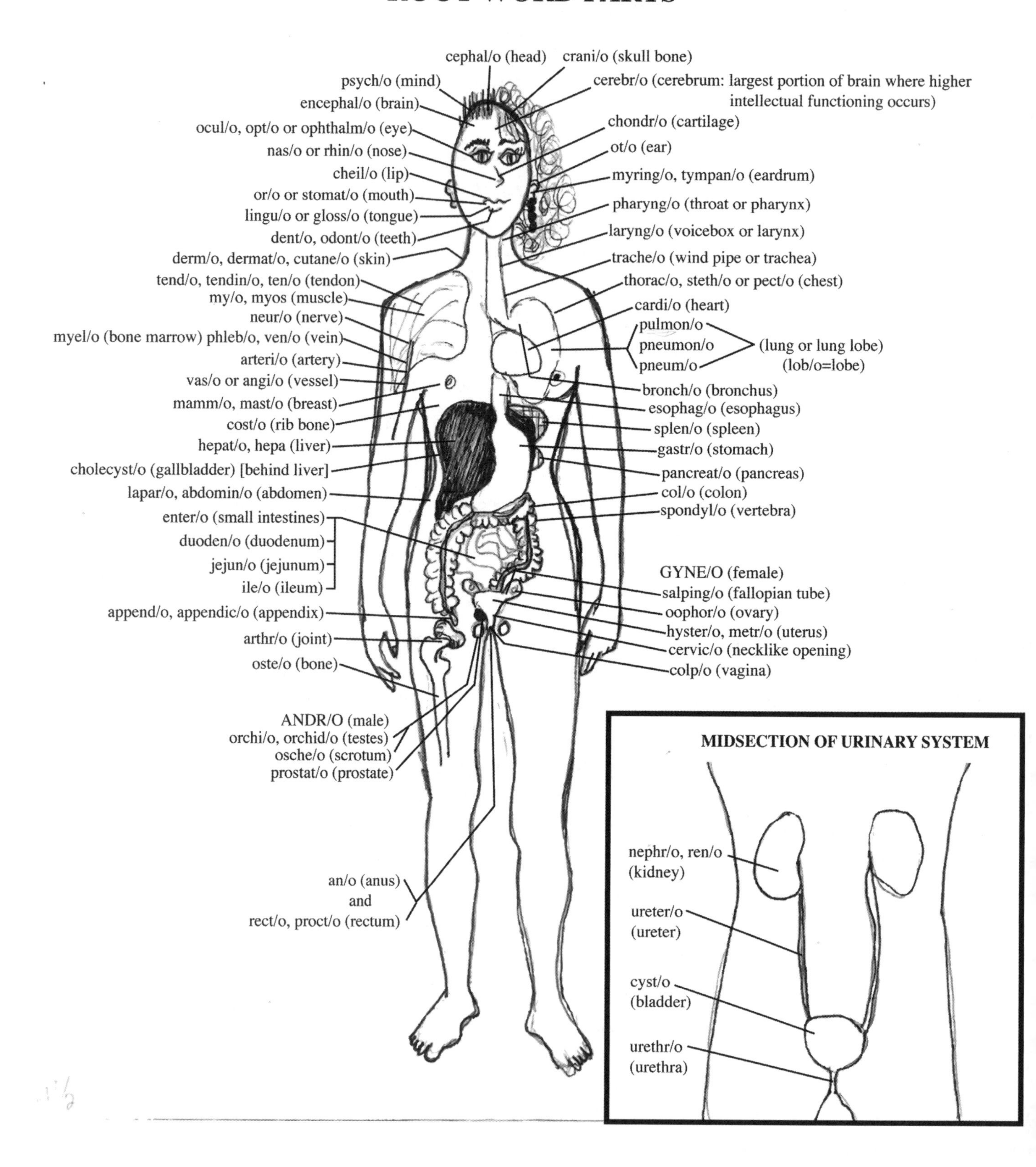

ROOT WORD PARTS

(usually end in a "/o" to let you know that this is a root word part and that another word part needs to be added to create a complete medical term. The "/o" is only a symbol noting a root part and must be dropped prior to adding a suffix). Occasionally "/o" is also used to combine forms.

• Andrology = a medical term defined as the process or procedure of studying a male body
(root word part: andr/o)
• Gynecology = a medical term defined as the process or procedure of studying a female body
(root word part: gynec/o)

PRACTICE, PRACTICE, PRACTICE...

Exercise 1:

As soon as you have received new medical terms, begin to review. Using blank 3" X 5" index cards, create flashcards to review all of the new medical terms in this chapter by writing each of the correctly spelled terms five times on one side of the index card and the definition of each term on the other side of the index card. Keeping all of these cards in your right pocket, continually review all of the cards throughout the day. Whenever you have learned a card, place it in your left pocket. After you have learned all of these new terms, periodically refresh your memory with review.

Exercise 2:

Create a chapter study guide that incorporates all of the root word parts presented on the last two pages, adds another element (a suffix or ending word part of medical term), and then builds a list of medical terms you'll need to know. It's like putting a slice of bread (the suffix) under a piece of meat (the root word part). Now you have a sandwich you can eat (a medical term you can use in a sentence). A root word part plus a suffix equals or makes a medical term.

For example:

a root word part (dermat/o meaning skin) + a suffix (-itis meaning inflammation of)
= a medical term (dermatitis)

OR

a root word part (splen/o meaning spleen) + a suffix (-ectomy meaning the process or procedure of surgical removal or excision of)
= a medical term (splenectomy) - meaning the process or procedure of surgical removal of the spleen

OR

a root word part (ot/o meaning ear) + a suffix (-ology meaning the process or procedure of science or study)
= a medical term (otology) - meaning the process or procedure of science or study of the ear

To complete this exercise and to have the study guide, you'll need to make a list of medical terms by adding the suffixes -itis and -ectomy to all of the root word parts on the last two pages. Some of these terms are rare or even silly. However, the idea is just to practice making medical terms.

Exercise 3:

Spelling. Taking the top ten toughest medical terms to spell, trace the correct spelling on a textured surface. For example: pour salt or sugar on a table then use your index finger to trace the correct spelling for each of the ten medical terms. After you've practiced repeatedly spelling these terms, clean up.

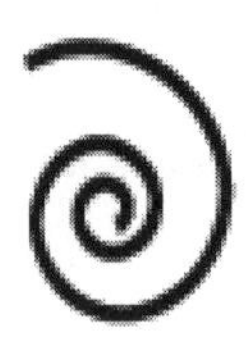

Chapter 2

Specialists and Specialties Terms:

Once you have these 'building materials', you are armed with the tools to begin to 'divide and conquer' new and less familiar terms in the future. Medical terms, when divided, are made up from various word parts. By understanding these word parts, you will conquer medical terminology.

A prefix is a word part used at the beginning of a medical term. 'A-' is a prefix meaning 'without, no, or not any.' 'Febrile' is a medical term meaning 'fever'. When you put them together, you can make the new medical term: afebrile (without fever).

1 medical term = 1 prefix + 1 medical term or 1 root word part

afebrile = a- + febrile (maybe used as either a root or term)

Medical terms can be constructed in many different ways:

1 medical term = 1 (or more) prefixes
+
1 (or more) root word parts
+
1 (or more) suffixes

For example: asymptomatic = (a- prefix, meaning 'without,' symptomat/o, a root word part meaning 'sign,' and -ic, a suffix meaning 'related to').

There are many different ways to put together a medical term to be used in a sentence. **However; prefixes, root word parts, and suffixes are only parts of a word that when used alone cannot properly be used in a sentence.**

This chapter will focus upon the suffix, a word part used at the end of a medical term and generally added to a root word part. 'Bi/o' is a root word part meaning 'life or living cells'. '-olog' is a suffix meaning 'science or study of' and '-y' is a suffix meaning 'process or procedure of'. When you put them together, you can create the medical term 'biology'.

1 medical term = 1 root word part
+
1 (or more) suffixes

STUDY GUIDE:

MEDICAL TERMS	ROOT WORD PARTS	SUFFIXES
Biology =	bi- (life or living cells) +	-olog (study or science of)
Cardiology =	cardi- (heart)	
Nephrology =	nephr- (kidney)	
Psychology =	psych- (mind) +	-y (process or procedure of)
Cardiologist		-ist (specialist)
Nephrologist		
Psychologist		
Internist		
Orthopedist		OR
Psychiatrist		-iatrist (specialist)
Podiatrist	pod- (foot or feet)	OR
Physician		-ician (specialist)
Pediatrician		
Obstetrician		OR
Practitioner		-er (specialist)

MEDICAL TERM STUDY GUIDE & DEFINITIONS

SPECIALTY/ SPECIALIST

bariatrics/ bariatrician (weight specialist)
embryology/ embryologist (prenatal specialist)
endocrinology/ endocrinologist (ductless gland specialist)
epidemiology/ epidemiologist (disease study specialist)
geriatrics/ gerontologist (specialist on aging)
neonatology/ neonatologist (specialist in infants up to 6 weeks old)
nosology/ nosologist (specialist of systematic disease classification)
oncology/ oncologist (specialist on tumors)
pathology/ pathologist (morbid tissue specialist)
urology/ urologist (specialist of urinary and male reproductive issues)
acupressurist (specialist in an ancient Asian system of healing with therapeutic pressure)
acupuncturist (specialist in puncture to balance blocked meridians, chakras or energy pathways to promote healing)
alternative medicine (OR)
complimentary care (care focused upon restoring or facilitating health maintenance)
chiropractor (specialist in hand manipulation for treatment of musculoskeletal issues)
naturopath (specialist of natural treatment with diet, light, heat, cold, water, or vitamins)
massage therapist (soft tissue manipulation specialist who promotes healing and/ or health)

DECODING THE MYSTERY:

* Whenever you encounter a new medical term, try the 'divide and conquer' strategy starting at the back of the word then working your way forward. For example: salpingoophorectomy

- Step 1: Divide the new term into word parts
  (root + root + suffix):
  salping oophor ectomy

- Step 2: Working from the back of the new term, define
  each recognizable element (then look up the unfamiliar)

- Step 3: Translation: The process or procedure of surgical removal of ovaries and
  fallopian tubes = salpingoophorectomy

PRACTICE, PRACTICE, PRACTICE...

Exercise 1:

As soon as you have received new medical terms, begin to review. Using blank 3" X 5" index cards, create flashcards to review all of the new medical terms in this chapter by writing each of the correctly spelled terms five times on one side of the index card and the definition of each term on the other side of the index card. Keeping all of these cards in your right pocket, continually review all of the cards throughout the day. Whenever you have learned a card, place it in your left pocket. After you have learned all of these new terms, periodically refresh your memory with review.

Exercise 2:

Career Exploration.

1. I am a specialist of disorders related to the feet. Who am I? podiatrist
2. I am a specialist of issues related to weight. Who am I? bariatrician
3. I am a specialist in the science of children. Who am I? pediatrician
4. I am a specialist in inserting needles for realignment of chakra (or chi). Who am I? acupuncturist
5. I am a specialist in general physical medicine. Who am I? physician
6. I am a specialist in male reproductive issues. Who am I? urologist
7. I am a specialist in new growths, neoplasms, or tumors. Who am I? oncologist
8. I am a specialist in the study of morbid tissue . Who am I? pathologist
9. I am a specialist in the study of newborns up to 6 weeks. Who am I? neonatologist
10. I am a specialist in the study of disease. Who am I? epidemiologist

Exercise 3:

Word Scramble. Unscramble these letters representing the medical term for various specialists.

1. tomapightsollh= _ _ _ _ _ _ _ _ _ _ _ _ _ _ _ _ _ _
2. sgooslitn= _ _ _ _ _ _ _ _ _ _ _
3. ttpnoraahu= _ _ _ _ _ _ _ _ _ _ _
4. rrrpoicohcta= _ _ _ _ _ _ _ _ _ _ _ _ _ _
5. stodlironcoineg= _ _ _ _ _ _ _ _ _ _ _ _ _ _ _ _ _ _

ANSWER KEY: Exercise 2: 1) podiatrist, 2) bariatrician, 3) pediatrician, 4) acupuncturist, 5) physician, 6) urologist, 7) oncologist, 8) pathologist, 9) neonatologist, 10) epidemiologist

Exercise 3: 1) ophthalmologist, 2) nosologist, 3) naturopath, 4) chiropractor, 5) endocrinologist

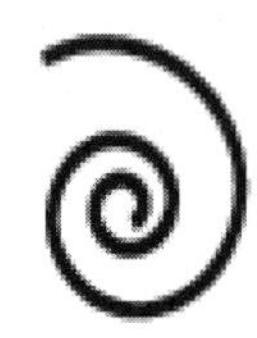

Chapter 3

Surgical Suffixes.

The suffix is a word part added to the end of a root word part to create a medical term. All of the suffixes presented in this chapter relate to different surgical procedures. Any of the new suffixes illustrated today may appear in various future combinations with any root word part from Chapter 1. Review, review, review.

STUDY GUIDE: SURGICAL SUFFIXES

SUFFIX/PRONOUNCIATION	DEFINITION	MEDICAL TERM
-ectomy (ek-to-me)	process or procedure: to excise or to surgically remove	tonsillectomy appendectomy
-cision (si-shun)	to cut, pertaining to in-, into ex-, out	incision excision
-desis (de-sis)	binding together	vasodesis
-otomy (ot-o-me)	process or procedure of cutting into or making an incision into	laparotomy colotomy tracheotomy
-ostomy (os-to-me)	process or procedure of artificially establishing a mouth-like opening	colostomy ileostomy tracheostomy
-orrhaphy (or-ra-fe)	process or procedure of surgical repair	nephrorrhaphy hysterorrhaphy
-opexy (o-pex-e)	process or procedure of fixing and suturing	salpingopexy hysteropexy cheilopexy
-oplasty (o-plas-te)	process or procedure of reconstructive surgery	rhinoplasty arthroplasty angioplasty
-otripsy (o-trip-se) (lith=stone)	process or procedure of crushing or destroying	neurotripsy osteotripsy lithotripsy
-ocentesis (sen-te-sis)	surgical puncture to remove, withdraw, or aspirate fluid	arthrocentesis amniocentesis

PRACTICE, PRACTICE, PRACTICE...

Exercise 1:

As soon as you have received new medical terms, begin to review. Using blank 3" X 5" index cards, create flashcards to review all of the new medical terms in this chapter by writing each of the correctly spelled terms five times on one side of the index card and the definition of each term on the other side of the index card. Keeping all of these cards in your right pocket, continually review all of the cards throughout the day. Whenever you have learned a card, place it in your left pocket. After you have learned all of these new terms, periodically refresh your memory with review.

Exercise 2:

The Translator. As a student of medical terminology, your job will be to translate surgical procedures into a single representative medical term. For example:

Surgical Procedure	Medical Term
1. Surgical repair of uterus =	hysterorrhaphy
2. Fix kidneys into place and suture =	nephoopexy
3. Artificially establish a tracheal opening =	tracheostomy
4. Incision into the abdomen =	laparotomy
5. Related to cutting out =	excision
6. Surgical removal of a tonsil =	tonsillectomy
7. Nose reconstruction =	rhinoplasty
8. Nerve crushing/ destruction =	neurotripsy
9. Puncture to remove joint fluid =	arthrocentesis
10. Vessel reconstruction =	angioplasty

Exercise 3:

Jeopardy. The category is surgical procedures. When a medical term for a surgical procedure is given, your objective is to reply with the definition of that medical term in the form of a question. Each correct response = 200 points. For example:

Medical Term	Reply/ Question
• Osteoplasty	"What is the process or procedure of bone reconstruction surgery?"
1. Incision	related to cutting into
2. Amniocentesis	puncture to remove fluid from the amniotic sac
3. Ileostomy	artificially establish a mouth-like opening into the ileum
4. Orchiopexy	fix testes into place and suture
5. Salpingorrhaphy	surgical repair of fallopian tube

ANSWER KEY: Exercise 2: 1) hysterorrhaphy, 2) nephropexy, 3) tracheostomy, 4) laparotomy or abdominotomy, 5) excision, 6) tonsillectomy, 7) rhinoplasty, 8) neurotripsy, 9) arthrocentesis, 10) angioplasty

Exercise 3: 1) What is a surgical procedure related to cutting into? 2) What is a surgical procedure involving puncture to remove amniotic fluid? 3) What is a surgical procedure of surgically establishing an opening into the ileum? 4)What is the surgical procedure of fixing and suturing the testes into place? 5) What is the surgical procedure to repair the fallopian tubes?`

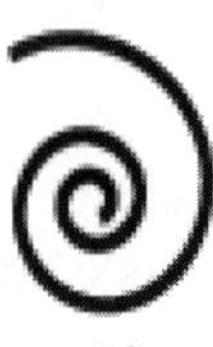

Chapter 4

Medical Suffixes: Symtoms and Conditions

STUDY GUIDE:

SUFFIX/PRONOUNCIATION	DEFINITION	MEDICAL TERM
-algia (al-ge-a) OR	pain, related to	neuralgia otalgia dentalgia
-odynia (o-din-e-a)	pain, related to	neurodynia abdominodynia
-cele (sel)	rupture or hernia	rectocele cystocele
-dipsia (dip-se-a)	thirst, related to (poly=excessive)	polydipsia
-drome (drom)	running together in a pattern (syn=symptoms united) (pro=preceeding or before)	syndrome prodromal
-ectasis (ek-ta-sis)	stretching, opening, or dilation	bronchiectasis
-emia (em-e-a)	related to, blood (an=without, no, not any)	anemia
-genesis (jen-e-sis)	production or origin (path=morbid tissue)	pathogenesis
-gnosis (gno-sis)	related to, knowledge (dia=thorough/pro=before)	diagnosis prognosis
-iasis (i-a-sis)	process of forming or presence (lith=stone)	lithiasis
-itis (i-tis)	inflammation of (hem=blood)	arthritis pharyngitis
-lysis (li-sis)	breaking down	hemolysis
-malacia (mal-a-se-a)	soften	osteomalacia
-megaly (meg-a-le)	process or procedure of enlarge-ment (-y=process)	cardiomegaly cystomegaly
-oid (oyd)	resembles or similar to (lip=fat) (muc=mucous) (thyr=shield) (xyph=dagger)	lipoid mucoid thyroid/xyphoid
-olysis (ol-i-sis)	destroy or separate (hem=blood)	hemolysis

SUFFIX/PRONOUNCIATION	DEFINITION	MEDICAL TERM
-oma (o-ma)	new growth, tumor, or neoplasm (lip=fat) (carcin=cancerous)	hematoma lipoma carcinoma
-opathy (o-path-e)	process or procedure of, any disease of (-y=process) (aden=gland)	adenopathy cardiomyopathy myopathy
-openia (o-pe-ne-a)	unusual reduction (leuk=white, as in WBC)	leukopenia
-orrhagia (or-rah-ge-a)	hemorrhage, related to	menorrhagia
-orrhea (or-re-a)	flow or discharge (py=bacteria or pus) (men=menstrual)	pyorrhea menorrhea
-osis (o-sis)	condition of	dermatosis neurosis
-paresis (par-e-sis)	remarkable weakness (hemi=half or one side)	hemiparesis
-phagia (fa-ge-a)	related to, eating or swallowing (a=without, no, not any)	aphagia
-phasia (fa-se-a)	related to, speech	aphasia
-plasia (pla-ze-a)	related to, cellular growth or development (hyper=excessive, hypo=low)	hyperplasia hypoplasia aplasia
-phonia (fo-ne-a)	related to, voice (due to a laryngeal issue)	aphonia
-plegia (pla-ge-a)	related to, paralysis (quad=four)	hemiplegia quadriplegia
-pnea (p-ne-a)	breathing (dys=difficult, painful)	apnea dyspnea
-ptosis (p-to-sis)	drooping (bleph=eyelid)	blephptosis
-rrhexis (rex-is)	rupture	colorrhexis
-spasm (spa-zm)	contraction or twitch (involuntary)	bronchospasm
-trophy (tro-fe)	process or procedure of development (from usage) (-y=process)	atrophy hypertrophy
-uria (yur)	urine or urination, related to	pyuria hematuria

PRACTICE, PRACTICE, PRACTICE...

Exercise 1:

As soon as you have received new medical terms, begin to review. Using blank 3" X 5" index cards, create flashcards to review all of the new medical terms in this chapter by writing each of the correctly spelled terms five times on one side of the index card and the definition of each term on the other side of the index card. Keeping all of these cards in your right pocket, continually review all of the cards throughout the day. Whenever you have learned a card, place it in your left pocket. After you have learned all of these new terms, periodically refresh your memory with review.

Exercise 2:

Without what? In this practice exercise, complete the blank with the appropriate medical term.

1. A- (without) + breathing = apnea
2. A- + voice = aphonia
3. A- + development = aplasia (cellular), atrophy (muscular)
4. A- + eating or swallowing = aphagia
5. A- + speech = aphasia

Exercise 3:

Walk and Talk. While walking, talk out silly new connections or ways to remember the new medical terms in this chapter (pneumonic tips). After about ten minutes of walking, jot down your ideas about how you could remember new terms. For example, gross or funny details tend to be more memorable. When I want to remember the term 'pyorrhea', I say it out loud to hear that it sounds like 'diarrhea' (flowing out of feces). Therefore, it may remind you that 'pyorrhea' stands for an image of flowing out of a bacteria filled pie (a silly mental picture to remember what 'py' represents).

While walking and talking; mentally picture the medical terms:

hemiparesis
hemiplegia
prodromal
prognosis
dermopathy, dentalgia, etc.
hematoma
lipoma
mucoid
hypertrophy
hyperplasia.

Be prepared to informally share your original review tips with the class and hand in your findings next class.

ANSWER KEY: Exercise 2: 1) apnea, 2) aphonia, 3) atrophy, 4) aphagia, 5) aphasia

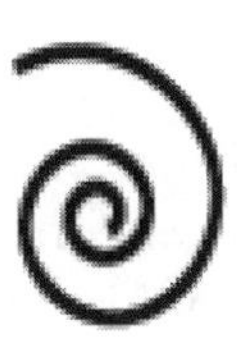

Chapter 5

Medical Suffixes: Instruments and Use.

STUDY GUIDE:

SUFFIX/PRONOUNCIATION	DEFINITION	MEDICAL TERM
-tome (tom)	instrument used for making thin slices	dermatome osteotome
-tomy (tom-e)	process or procedure of using an instrument to make thin slices	dermatomy osteotomy
-graph (graf)	instrument that records visually	radiograph electrocardiograph
-graphy (graf-e)	process or procedure of using an instrument to record visually	radiography electrocardiography angiography sonography
-gram (gram)	the product of using a recording instrument: the recording or image produced	mammogram sonogram radiogram angiogram
-ometer (om-et-er)	a measuring instrument	thermometer spirometer
-ometry (om-e-tre)	process or procedure of using a measuring instrument	pelvimetry thermometry spirometry
-oscope (o-skop)	instrument used for examining (usually visually OR by sound)	ophthalmoscope cystoscope arthroscope stethoscope fetoscope
-oscopy (o-skop-e)	process or procedure of using an instrument to examine	ophthalmoscopy cystoscopy fetoscopy

PRACTICE, PRACTICE, PRACTICE...

Exercise 1:

As soon as you have received new medical terms, begin to review. Using blank 3" X 5" index cards, creat flashcards to review all of the new medical terms in this chapter by writing each of the correctly spelled terms fiv times on one side of the index card and the definition of each term on the other side of the index card. Keepin all of these cards in your right pocket, continually review all of the cards throughout the day. Whenever you hav learned a card, place it in your left pocket. After you have learned all of these new terms, periodically refresh you memory with review.

Exercise 2:

Name That. Write the six medical terms that represent the instrument, process of using that instrument, an product (picture or recording) produced from using that instrument for ultrasound and x-ray.

Exercise 3:

Tuning into Clues. Carefully listening to new medical terms can be another useful decoding tool to determine term meaning. 'Scope, an instrument used to examine, sounds like 'soap'. How do the meaning and sound change when the 'e' becomes replaced by a 'y'?

ANSWER KEY: Exercise 2: 1) sonograph, 2) sonography, 3) sonogram, 4) radiograph, 5) radiography, 6) radiogram

Exercise 3: -scopy. The meaning changes to the process or procedure of using an instrument to examine. The sound changes to sound like 'soapie' (or so-pe).

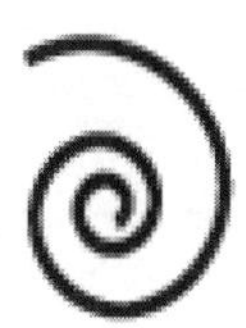

Chapter 6

Medical Prefixes: General, Amounts,Colors, Singulars and Plurals.

STUDY GUIDE:

PREFIX/PRONOUNCIATION	DEFINITION	MEDICAL TERM
a- (a), an-, or ar-	without, no, not any (febrile=fever)	afebrile
an- (an)	(-esthesia=feeling)	anesthesia
ar- (ar)	(-rhythmia=related to rhythm)	arrhythmia
	(-septic=related to contamination)	aseptic
	(-trophy=process of development)	atrophy
	(-pnea=breathing)	apnea
ab- (ab)	move away from	abduction
ad- (ad)	move toward or near	adduction
anti- (an-te)	against	antibiotic
bio- (bi-o)	life or living cells	biology
		bioethics
brady- (bra-de)	slow (-cardia=heart rate)	bradycardia
tachy- (tak-e)	fast	tachycardia
contra- (kon-tra)	against (indication=recommendation)	contraindication
de- (de)	remove or take away (hydrate=fluid input)	dehydrate
dia- (di-a)	running through	diarrhea
dys- (dis)	difficult or painful (-uria=urine)	dysuria
	(-pnea=breathing)	dyspnea
	(-phoria=related to mood)	dysphoria
	(trophy=process of development)	dystrophy
dis- (dis)	away from	disease
eu- (ew)	good or easy	euphoria
hemat- (he-mat)	blood	hematuria
	(-oma=new growth or tumor)	hematoma
hydr- (hi-dra)	fluids, liquids	hydrate
inter- (in-ter)	between	interaction
intra- (in-tra)	within	intramuscular
lip- (lip)	fat or fatty	lipoma
	(-oid=resembling or similar to)	lipoid
lith- (lith)	stone, stones (-osis=condition of)	lithosis
mal- (mal)	bad, poor, ill	malaise
	(occlusion=alignment)	malocclusion
noct- (nokt) OR nyct (nikt)	night, needing to get up at	nocturia
	nighttime	nycturia

PREFIX/PRONOUNCIATION	DEFINITION	MEDICAL TERM
necr- (nekr)	dead (-osis=condition of)	necrosis
pan- (pan)	all inclusive	pandemic
poly- (pol-e)	excessive, much (-uria=related to urine or urination)	polyuria
pre- (pre)	before	preoperative
post- (post)	after	postoperative
pro- (pro)	preceeding, early (-drom=signs)	prodromal
sclera- (skler)	hardening (-osis=condition of)	sclerosis
soma- (so-ma)	body (-ic=related to)	somatic
	(related to mind and body)	psychosomatic
sym- (sim)	united, together (signs)	symptom
or syn- (sin)	(-drome- symptoms united in a pattern)	syndrome
AMOUNTS		
nulli (nul-le)	zero or none (-para-live birth)	nullipara
hemi- (hem-e)	half, one side	hemisphere
	(-paresis=marked weakness)	hemiparesis
primi- (pre-me)	one, first	primipara
uni- (yu-ne)	one (lateral=related to side	unilateral
bi- (bi)	two or both (also, life)	biweekly
tri- (tri)	three	triweekly
quadri- (kwad-ri)	four (limbs) (-plegia=related to paralysis)	quadriplegia
multi- (mul-te)	many, multiple	multipara
semi- (sem-e)	partially	semicomatose
ipsi- (ip-se)	same	ipsilateral
hyper- (hi-per)	too much, above, or high	hyperactive
	(amount or location)	hypergastric hyperthyroid
	(high blood pressure)	hypertension
	(-glycemia=related to blood glucose)	hyperglycemia
hypo- (hi-po)	too little, not enough, or low	hypoactive
COLORS		
rub- (rewb) or eryth- (erith)	red (measles) or redness	rubella or erythema
alb- (alb)	white	albinism
melan- (mel-an)	black (-oma=new growth, tumor)	melanoma

PREFIX/PRONOUNCIATION	DEFINITION	MEDICAL TERM
cyan- (si-an)	blue (-osis=codition of)	cyanosis
cirrh- (sir)	orangish yellow (-osis=condition)	cirrhosis
poli- (po-le)	grey	poliomyelitis
xanth- (zanth)	yellow	xanthoderma

COMMON SINGULAR/PLURALS

SINGULAR	*(EXAMPLE)*	PLURAL	*(EXAMPLE)*
-a	*vertebra (bone in spinal column)*	-ae	*vertebrae*
-um	*ovum (egg)*	-a	*ova*
-us	*thrombus (blood clot)*	-i	*thrombi*
-is	*diagnosis (condition of thorough knowledge)*	-es	*diagnoses*
-ix	*appendix (appendage to large colon)*	-ices	*appendices*
-ma	*carcinoma (cancerous tumor)*	-mata	*carcinomata*
-inx	*meninx (membranes of brain and spinal cord)*	-inges	*meninges*
-anx	*phalanx (digit)*	-anges	*phalanges*
-en	*lumen (hollow tube opening)*	-ina	*lumina*

don't need to know

PRACTICE, PRACTICE, PRACTICE...

Exercise 1:

As soon as you have received new medical terms, begin to review. Using blank 3" X 5" index cards, creat flashcards to review all of the new medical terms in this chapter by writing each of the correctly spelled terms fiv times on one side of the index card and the definition of each term on the other side of the index card. Keepin all of these cards in your right pocket, continually review all of the cards throughout the day. Whenever you hav learned a card, place it in your left pocket. After you have learned all of these new terms, periodically refresh you memory with review.

Exercise 2:

Divide and Conquer. Divide the following TWO of each of these terms to create ONE new term of each. Do th math:

Singular Medical Term

1. 2 carcinomata divided by 1 = ______
2. 2 thrombi divided by 1 = ______
3. 2 lumina divided by 1 = ______
4. 2 phalanges divided by 1 = ______
5. 2 emboli divided by 1 = ______

Exercise 3: Cooperative Class Group Exercise:

The 'Dys-' Family. Some families are dysfunctional and difficult but this prefix can be easily conquered. List ALL of the possible medical terms with the prefix 'dys' and their meanings. Then, mingle as a class group and review chapter terms but switch to a different study partner every 1-2 minutes.

ANSWER KEY: Exercise 2: 1) carcinoma, 2) thrombus, 3) lumen, 4) phalanx, 5) embolus
Exercise 3: Dysuria, dyspnea, dysphoria, dystrophy, dyscardia, etc.

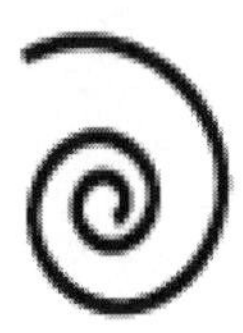

Chapter 7

Location, Location, Location.

STUDY GUIDE:

PREFIX/PRONOUNCIATION	DEFINITION	MEDICAL TERM
circum- (sir-kum)	around (-cise=cut)	circumcision
dextro- (dex-tro)	right (-rotation=turn)	dextrorotation
endo- (en-do)	inside, within (-scope=instrument used to examine)	endoscope
ecto- (ek-to)	outside of (-ic=related to) (top-=position in uterus)	ectopic
exo- (x-o)	outside	exogenous
extra- (x-tra)	outside	extrauterine
epi- (ep-e)	above or upon	epigastric
infra- (in-fra)	under (stern-=breast bone)	infrasternal
meta- (met-a)	beyond, change	metastasis
	or transformation (stasis=sameness)	metabolism
peri- (per-e)	around, surround	pericardium
	(related to outer edge)	peripheral
retro- (re-tro)	behind, back (related to turning)	retroversion
sinistro- (sin-is-tro)	left	sinistrorotation
trans- (tranz)	across, through	transvaginal
	(-verse=a dividing line)	transverse

MEDICAL TERMS	DEFINITIONS
anterior (or ventral) (A)	front, toward front
posterior (or dorsal) (P)	back, toward the rear
superior (or cephalic)	above (related toward head)
inferior (or caudal)	below
proximal	nearest to point of reference or attachment
distal	farther from point of reference or attachment
cephalic	head, related to
caudal	spine, related to
medial (or midline)	middle, related to
oblique	at an angle
lateral	side, related to

MEDICAL TERMS	DEFINITIONS
bilateral	both sides, related to
decubitus (or recumbent)	lying down, position of
Fowler's	sitting up, position of (enables easier respirations)
Trendelenburg	legs elevated higher than heart, position of (increases venous return)
sagittal	a vertical body plane, related to
midsagittal	a vertical body plane in the middle of the body (equally divides right and left sides of body)
coronal	a vertical body plane that divides the body between anterior and posterior, related to
transverse	a horizonal body plane that divides the body across between superior and inferior
quadrants	four anterior divisions of the abdomen, identified from patient's perspective: R.U.Q.,L.U.Q.,L.L.Q.,R.L.Q. (right lower quadrant)

BODY PLANES

- coronal plane - an imaginary division between anterior and posterior aspects of the body
- mid saggital plane - an imaginary division between right and left sides of the body
- transverse plane - an imaginary division across or through between superior and inferior portions of the body

PRACTICE, PRACTICE, PRACTICE...

Exercise 1:

As soon as you have received new medical terms, begin to review. Using blank 3" X 5" index cards, create flashcards to review all of the new medical terms in this chapter by writing each of the correctly spelled terms five times on one side of the index card and the definition of each term on the other side of the index card. Keeping all of these cards in your right pocket, continually review all of the cards throughout the day. Whenever you have learned a card, place it in your left pocket. After you have learned all of these new terms, periodically refresh your memory with review.

Exercise 2:

Like Simon, Sam Says. As an individual or classroom group, follow ONLY what Sam says. Anyone who does not do what Sam says will sit out the rest of the game and be subject to silly sanctions.

1. Sam says 'assume Fowler's position'.
2. Sam says 'stretch your caudal region'.
3. Sam says 'illustrate a cephalic erection'.
4. 'Relax'.
5. Sam says 'relax'.
6. Sam says 'point to your epigastric area'.
7. Sam says 'stand up and dextrorotate your body like a ballerina'.
8. 'Sit down'.

9. Sam says ‘stop then sinistrorotate like a dolphin’
10. Sam says ‘relax and sit down’.

Exercise 3:

Comical Choreography. This exercise may be practiced as an individual but is more fun to practice as a synchronized classroom group. You are to go to the front of the room and move anteriorly to the rest of the room. You are to move your leg distally to the salute position then assume a proximal leg position. Hop on one foot for 5 seconds then rest. Safely illustrate your superior position to an identified inferior object. Then, physically illustrate your understanding of the transverse, coronal, and midsaggital planes then the quadrants.

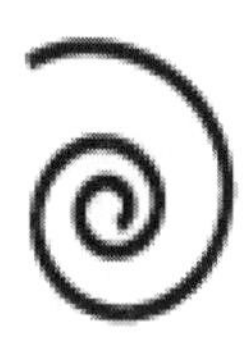

Chapter 8

Miscellaneous Foundation Terms

STUDY GUIDE:

MEDICAL TERMS	PRONOUNCIATIONS	DEFINITIONS
abdomen	(ab-do-men)	general area from lower ribs to pubis
abdominal	(ab-dom-in-al)	related to the abdomen
abortion	(a-bor-shun)	pregnancy termination
abscess	(ab-ses)	a localized collection or nodule of bacteria under a surface
acute	(a-kut)	a short term illness with a sudden onset and severe sx (symptoms)
chronic	(kron-ik)	a long term illness with slow onset and familiar sx (symptoms)
adhesion	(ad-he-shun)	fibrous scar tissue that tends to form in an unruly manner
afebrile	(a-fe-bril)	without fever
febrile	(fe-bril)	fever
axilla	(ak-sil-la)	armpit
anomaly	(a-nom-a-le)	abnormality
biopsy	(bi-op-se)	procedure for examining life or living tissue
catheter	(kath-et-er)	a flexible, plastic tube (often for fluid passage)
communicable	(com-mun-ik-ab-el)	contagious
congenital	(kon-jen-it-al)	present at birth
hereditary	(her-ed-i-tar-e)	present at conception
continence	(kon-tin-enz)	ability to control urine or feces
constrict	(kon-strikt)	narrow
dilate	(di-lat)	widen
edema	(ed-em-a)	swelling
emesis	(em-e-sis)	vomit
embolus	(em-bo-lus)	a free-floating clot of blood, air, fat, bacteria, or foreign body that may lodge
thrombus	(throm-bus)	a stationary blood clot
etiology	(et-e-ol-og-e)	process of studying cause
exacerbation	(x-a-ser-ba-shun)	worsening or returning of symptoms
hemorrhage	(hem-or-aj)	sudden onset of profuse bleeding
hemostasis	(he-mo-sta-sis)	controlled bleeding
hepatorrhexis	(he-pat-or-x-is)	liver rupture

MEDICAL TERMS	PRONOUNCIATIONS	DEFINITIONS
homeostasis	(hom-e-o-sta-sis)	the body's maintenance of internal balance (temperature, pulse, respiration, cell division rate, and hormonal levels) at rest
iatrogenic	(i-at-ro-gen-ik)	side effect or response to a physician's treatment
icterus	(ik-ter-us)	jaundice
idiopathic	(id-e-o-path-ik)	no known cause
incontinence	(in-kon-tin-ens)	inability to control urine or feces
introitus	(in-troy-tus)	vaginal cavity
ischemia	(is-ke-me-a)	insufficient blood/oxygen supply
leukopenia	(loo-k-o-pen-e-a)	related to a low or insufficient white blood cell count
lipopenia	(lip-o-pen-e-a)	related to low or insufficient lipids
lumen	(lu-men)	hollow tube opening or passage
meatus	(me-a-tus)	opening or passage, such as urinary opening
metabolism	(met-ab-o-lizm)	the process by which all ingested nourishment is converted to heat or other energy
metastasis	(met-as-ta-sis)	spread beyond original site
nosocomial	(nos-o-ko-me-al)	caused by exposure within a treatment facility
orifice	(or-if-is)	a body cavity entrance (for example, anal or oral)
os	(os)	mouth or mouthlike opening (for example, cervical)
osteoblast	(os-te-o-blast)	a bone forming cell
oligdipsia	(o-lig-dip-se-a)	related to little or scanty thirst
palliative	(pal-e-a-tiv)	related to soothing care focused only on comfort
palpable	(pal-pa-bul)	ability to gently feel
palpate	(pal-pat)	to gently feel
patent	(pa-tent)	open or unblocked (for example, airway or lumen)
perforation	(per-for-a-shun)	hole
perineum	(per-i-ne-um)	the area between the genitals and the anus
placebo	(pla-se-bo)	a neutral substance used to test drug effectiveness
pleural	(pler-al)	related to membranes of the chest cavity linings

MEDICAL TERMS	PRONOUNCIATIONS	DEFINITIONS
prolapse	(pro-laps)	flopping out of place, displacement
prophylaxis	(pro-fil-ak-sis)	preventative
purulent	(pur-u-lent)	bacterial
remission	(re-mis-shun)	temporary symptom cessation
sequela	(se-kwel-a)	a pathological condition from a previous disease, attack, or injury
serous	(se-rus)	pinkish-yellowish fluid from blood
somatic	(so-mat-ik)	related to the body
sputum	(spu-tum)	lung production, what is coughed up
tolerance	(tol-er-anz)	the need to ingest more of an agent to achieve the originally sought effect
titration/titrate	(ti-tra-shun)	a measured increase of a solution is added to a known amount of solution in order to achieve the calculation of a complete interaction or optimal dosage for an individual
triage	(tre-aj)	a prioritization system based upon medical urgency
tumescence/tumescent	(tu-mes-sens)	swelling
viscera	(vis-er-a)	internal abdominal organs
visceroptosis	(vis-er-op-to-sis)	visceral displacement
void	(voyd)	urinate

WHAT'S THE DIFFERENCE?

aphagia	aphasia	aphonia	aphoria
dysphagia	dysphasia	dysphonia	dysphoria
polyphagia	polyphasia	polyphonia	polyphoria
tachyphagia	tachyphasia	tachyphonia	tachyphoria
bradyphagia	bradyphasia	bradyphonia	bradyphoria

aphagia	without eating or swallowing
dysphagia	difficult or painful eating or swallowing
polyphagia	excessive or much eating or swallowing
tachyphagia	~~excessive or~~ fast eating or swallowing
bradyphagia	~~excessive or~~ slow eating or swallowing
aphasia	~~excessive or~~ without speech
dysphasia	~~excessive or~~ difficult or painful speech
polyphasia	excessive or much speech
tachyphasia	fast speech
bradyphasia	slow speech

aplasia - no cellular growth or development

aphonia	without voice (due to a laryngeal issue)
dysphonia	difficult or painful voice (due to a laryngeal issue)
aphoria	without mood
dysphoria	difficult or painful mood
polyphoria	excessive mood
tachyphoria	fast moodiness ↑ change of moods
bradyphoria	slow moodiness ↓ change of moods
polyphonia	excessive or much voice (due to a laryngeal issue)
tachyphonia	fast voice (due to a laryngeal issue)
bradyphonia	slow voice (due to a laryngeal issue)

PRACTICE, PRACTICE, PRACTICE........

Exercise 1:

As soon as you have received new medical terms, begin to review. Using black 3"X5" index cards, create flashcards to review all of the new medical terms in this chapter by writing each of the correctly spelled terms five times on one side of the index card and the definition of each term on the other side of the index card. Keeping all of these cards in your right pocket, continually review all of the cards throughout the day. Wheneve you have learned a card, place it in your left pocket. After you have learned all of these new terms, periodically refresh your memory with review.

Exercise 2:

Medical Term Hangman. With a partner, review the medical term definition as well as the number of blanks provided. Your partner peeks at the answer key (on the next page) and monitors whether your letter guess is correct or not. You are to state and write in your guess as to what letters will complete in the blanks provided in order to complete the correctly spelled medical term that best corresponds to the definition provided. For each incorrect letter guess, you must draw a portion of a hangman. One incorrect letter guess equals the drawing of either an arm, a trunk, a leg, a head, a foot, a hand, an eye, a nose, hair, or a mouth. If a hangman becomes fully drawn, review Exercise 1.

HANGMAN DRAWING	MEDICAL TERM LETTERS	DEFINITION
1)	_ _ _ _ _ _	vomit
2)	_ _ _ _ _ _ _ _ _	difficult speech
3)	_ _ _ _ _ _ _	a free floating clot
4)	_ _ _ _ _	swelling
5)	_ _ _ _ _ _ _ _ _ _	related to a side effect
6)	_ _ _ _ _ _ _	without swallowing ability

) _ _ _ _ _ _ _ _ _ _ _ _ a hole

) _ _ _ _ _ _ _ _ _ _ _ related to unknown cause

) _ _ _ _ _ _ open, not blocked

0) _ _ _ _ _ _ _ _ _ process of studying cause

Exercise 3:

Fingerpaint a term. For any medical terms that are particularly challenging for you to spell; finger paint the spelling on a smooth washable surface with paint, pudding, whipped cream, or sand. Fingerpaint each term ten times.

ANSWER KEY: 1) emesis, 2) aphasia, 3) embolus, 4) edema, 5) iatrogenic, 6) aphagia, 7) perforation, 8) idiopathic, 9) patent, 10) etiology

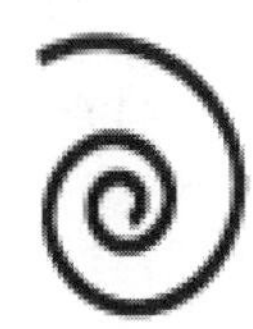

Chapter 9

Basic Diagnostics and Abbreviations

STUDY GUIDE:

ABBREVIATIONS	DEFINITIONS/IMAGING TECHNIQUES
C.A.T., C.T., or C.T.S. (ionizing imaging)	computerized axial tomography, x-ray series taken from a full circular rotation that pinpoints radiographic beam and surveys transverse planes of tissue to produce an absorption analysis that precisely reconstructs the image of focus (offers a better illustration of the axes and relationships of structures than a radiogram or x-ray)
M.R.I. (nonionizing imaging)	magnetic resonance imaging: a diagnostic radiogram using electromagnetic energy providing brain, soft tissue and musculoskeletal images. By using a radiofrequency pulse, absorption of energy is caused and released that then transforms to an image after this energy current passes through a radiofrequency receiver (contraindicated for patients with pacemakers or ferromagnetic aneurismal clips/devices)
P.E.T.	positron emission tomography: detects cancer and dementia by injecting the patient with radioactive sugar that illustrates 'hotspots' (where the sugar burns faster due to a presence of a tumor)
C.X.R.	chest x-ray

- Ionizing imaging is a process of producing pictures with radiation. Nonionizing imaging produces images without radiation or its potential side effects.
- Radiography is a process form of ionzing imaging in which a radiograph (or x-ray machine) radiation from x-rays pass through the body site to produce images or radiograms (x-ray pictures).
- Contrast medium is an internal substance utilized to clearly delineate anatomical structures or sites. For example: barium, air, or carbon dioxide.
- Nuclear Medicine Imaging (or Radionuclide Organ Imaging) is the process of injecting or ingesting radioactive isotopes designed to emit gamma rays that are recorded by a camera that produces images showing the gamma ray location. These pictures are helpful for showing the size, shape, location, and function of body organs.
- Sonography is the diagnostic procedure of producing images using ultrasound (u/s, us, or sound waves). A transducer (a device used to scan in order to visualize a tissue) uses high frequency sound waves to visualize dense structure reflections that provide moving images on a monitor. Abdominal sites, fetuses, cardiovascular sites, and glands are frequently imaged.

S.O.A.P.I.E. Organization of Information Format

Subjective entries: what the patient stated (pt. c/o otalgia)

Objective entries: objective information gathered (T101.2F, TM erythematous)

Assessment: given all of the subjective and objective information, the diagnosis is made (BOM)

Plan: recommended course of treatment (Augmentin, 500mg, po, BID, x 10 days)

Intervention: what was actually done (all medication given, as directed)

Evaluation: was the intervention successful? (both ears rechecked and unremarkable). Yes.

STUDY GUIDE:

ABBREVIATIONS	DEFINITIONS
Dx or Bx	diagnosis or biopsy
Hx or H&P	history - remarkable past physical & psychological
Rx, Tr, or Tx	prescription or recipe, treatment, traction, or transfer
Sx	symptoms or surgery
CC	chief complaint or predominant concern
c	with
c/o	complains of (patient's reason for the visit)
r/o	rule out or differential diagnosis
y/o	years old (age)
FH or SH	family history or social history
PH or OH	past history or occupational history
sg	physical signs
Lx	lumpectomy
Mx	mastectomy
A.I.D.S	acquired immune deficiency syndrome
A.R.C.	A.I.D.S.-related complex
A.D.R.	adverse drug reaction
C.A.	carcinoma
C.H.D.	coronary heart disease
C.H.F.	congestive heart failure
C.O.L.D. or C.O.P.D.	chronic obstructive lung disease (or pulmonary disease)
C.P.	cerebral palsy
C.P.R.	cardiopulmonary resuscitation
C.V.A. or C.V.D.	cerebrovascular accident or cardiovascular disease
CXR	chest x-ray
D/C or dc	discontinue or discharge
D.J.D.	degenerative joint disease
D.N.R.	do not resuscitate

ABBREVIATIONS	DEFINITIONS
D.O.B.	date of birth
D.S.B.	drug seeking behavior
D.V.T.	deep vein thrombosis
F.B.	foreign body
F.U.O.	fever of unknown (or undetermined) origin
G.C.	gonorrhea
G.C.P.	good clinical practice
G.S.W.	gunshot wound
H.P.V.	human papilloma virus
H.R.T.	hormone replacement therapy
I&O or I.M.P.	intake and output record for 24 hours or impression
M.D.	muscular dystrophy or medical doctor
M.I.	myocardial infarction
M.S.	multiple sclerosis
N.B.M.	nothing by mouth
N.P.O.	nothing per os or nothing by mouth
N.K.A. or N.K.D.A.	no known allergies or no known drug allergies
N.S.A.I.D.	non-steroidal anti-inflammatory drug
N.T.D. or N.A.D.	neural tube defect or no acute distress
O2	oxygen
O.D.	overdose
O.T.C.	over the counter
P or pt. or P.E.	pulse or patient or physical exam
P.I.D. or P.I.	pelvic inflammatory disease or present illness
P.R.N. or P.M.H.	as needed or post medical history
R or RRR	respirations or rectally or regular rate & rhythm
R.A. or R.O.S. (or SR)	rheumatoid arthritis or review of sx (systems review)
S	without or subjective (what the pt. states)
S.O.B.	shortness of breath
S.O.S.	if necessary
STAT	immediately
S.T.D.	sexually transmitted disease
T	temperature
T&A	tonsillectomy and adenoidectomy
T.I.A.	transient ischemic attack (mini-stroke)
L.L.Q. or U.L.Q.	lower left quadrant or upper left quadrant
U.R.I.	upper respiratory infection
U.R.Q. or L.R.Q.	upper right quadrant or lower right quadrant
U/S or U.C.H.D.	ultrasound or usual childhood diseases
U.T.I. or V.S.	urinary tract infection or vital signs T, P, R, PR, B/P

ABBREVIATIONS	DEFINITIONS
W.N.L. or WDWN	within normal limits or well developed & nourished
a.t.c.	around the clock
q or Q	every
q.d.	every day
q.o.d.	every other day
q.h.	every hour
q2h	every 2 hours
q3h	every 3 hours
q4h	every 4 hours
b.i.d.	twice daily (for example: 8a.m. and 8p.m.)
t.i.d.	three times daily (for example: 8a.m., 2p.m., and 8p.m.)
q.i.d.	four times daily (for example: 8a.m., 12n, 4p.m., & 8p.m.)
h.s.	hours of sleep or at bedtime
a.c.	before meals
p.c.	after meals
p.r.n.	as needed
ad lib	as desired
stat	immediately

ABBREVIATIONS	DEFINITIONS / ROUTES OR TYPES OF ADMINISTRATION
P.O.	by mouth or per os
S.L.	sublinqually or under the tongue
S.Q.	subcutaneous
I.D.	intradermal
I.M.	intramuscular
I.V.	intravenous
R.	by rectum or rectally
F.S.A.	flexible savings account for health care costs that accumulate on a pre-tax basis (but are forfeited if unused in a year)
H.D.H.P.	minimal deductibles of approximately $1,000. annually with less expensive premiums as a health plan
H.R.A.	health care reimbursement accounts and medical expense savings that can be rolled over annually
H.S.A.	health savings account: portable insurance policy (with a high deductible)

ABBREVIATIONS	DEFINITIONS / ROUTES OR TYPES OF ADMINISTRATION
H.M.O.	health maintenance organization: managed care plans with specific and limited options of facility locations & physicians
P.P.O.	preferred provider organization: offers 'preferred' networks with fee-for-service coverage (with greater choices than HMO)
W.P.	wellness program: company sponsored initiatives that encourage positive health behaviors (for example: exercise classes, weight reduction plans, stop smoking workshops, etc.)
LEGAL ABBREVIATIONS/TERMS	
A.M.A.	against medical advice
D.N.R.	a 'do not resuscitate' legal directive (despite physical need otherwise)
consent form	a permission for medical or surgical care (legal document signed by legal guardian or patient)

PHYSICAL EXAMINATION NOTES	
H.E.E.N.T.	head, eyes, ears, nose, and throat
P.E.R.L.A.	pupils equal and reactive to light accomodation
P.E.	physical exam
pt.	patient
S.O.A.P.I.E.	a note-taking format used for recording a physical exam: subjective, objective, assessment, plan, intervention, and evaluation

PRACTICE, PRACTICE, PRACTICE...

Exercise 1:

As soon as you have received new medical terms, begin to review. Using blank 3"X5" index cards, create flashcards to review all of the new medical terms in this chapter by writing each of the correctly spelled terms five times on one side of the index card and the definition of each term on the other side of the index card. Keeping all of these cards in your right pocket, continually review all of the cards throughout the day. Whenever you have learned a card, place it in your left pocket. After you have learned all of these new terms, periodically refresh your memory with review.

Exercise 2:

Get a Clue. Abbreviations are commonly spotted on physical exam notes. As a student of Medical Terminology, please translate the abbreviated clues in the following notes:

1) S: Pt. c/o L.R.Q. discomfort, nausea, and malaise.

2) O: T 100.8 F, P 80, R 18. L.R.Q. tenderness.

3) A: U/S L.R.Q., C.B.C. Dx: appendicitis

4) P: Appendectomy and Rx: Augmentin, 500mg. (p.o.), BID x10 days

5) I: Appendectomy and Rx completed.

6) E: Sx resolved.

7) Aspirin, grain 5, (p.o.) Q4h, p.r.n. for back pain.

8) Pt. c/o S.O.B., nausea, fatigue, and left shoulder discomfort. R/o M.I..

9) stat

10) 8 y/o c/o cough, fever, wheezing, and S.O.B.. CXR reveals acute bronchitis.

Exercise 3:

Cranium Crunch. Using a book marker; cover the left margin abbreviations read the definitions then give the abbreviations for each of these definitions. Remove the bookmarker in order to check your answers for accuracy.

ANSWER KEY: 1) Subjective: Patient complains of lower right abdominal quadrant discomfort, nausea, and malaise. 2) Objective: Temperature 100.8 degrees farenheit, pulse 80, respirations 18. Lower right quadrant tenderness. 3) Assessment: Ultrasound lower right quadrant. Complete blood count test. Diagnosis:inflammation of appendix. 4) Plan: procedure of surgical excision of appendix. Prescription: Augmentin (an antibiotic), 500mg. (dosage), (p.o. = by mouth), B.I.D. (twice daily) for a 10 day duration. 5) Done. 6) Symptoms resolved (cured) 7) Aspirin, 5 grains (dosage), (by mouth) every 4 hours, as needed for back pain. 8) Patient complains of shortness of breath, nausea, fatigue, and left shoulder discomfort. Rule out a myocardial infarction (heart attack). 9) immediately. 10) eight year old complains of cough, fever, wheezing, and shortness of breath. Chest x-ray reveals acute bronchial inflammation.

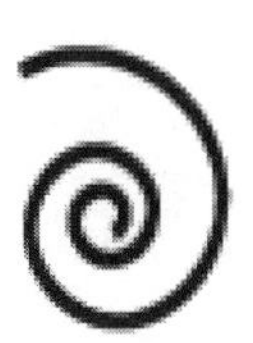

Chapter 10

Integumentary System
The integumentary system serves as a temperature regulator, protective covering, and waste disposal apparatus.

STUDY GUIDE:

ANATOMICAL TERMS	PRONOUNCIATIONS	DEFINITIONS
adipose	(ad-i-pos)	fat tissue
dermis	(der-mis)	middle skin layer (with sebaceous gland)
epidermis	(ep-i-der-mis)	top or outermost layer of skin
subcutaneous	(sub-ku-tan-e-us)	under the skin: adipose and blood vessels

DESCRIPTIVE TERMS	PRONOUNCIATIONS	DEFINITIONS
bulla	(bul-la)	blister (often large): skin lesion with clear fluid inside
vesicle	(ves-ik-el)	blister: skin lesion with clear fluid inside
pustule	(pus-chul)	skin lesion filled with bacteria
macule	(mak-yul)	any flat and discolored skin lesion
papule	(pap-ul)	any raised or elevated discolored skin lesion
nodule	(nod-ul)	any subcutaneously palpable lesion
cyst	(sist)	a moveable fluid-filled lesion
fissure	(fis-sur)	a surface crack in the skin
plaque	(plak)	silvery scales symptomatic of psoriasis
erosion	(e-ro-shun)	a tissue compromise/ wasting away of outer layer of skin
ulcer	(ul-ser)	a skin tissue compromise or destruction
perforation	(per-for-a-shun)	a hole
wheal	(wel)	a bleb or bubble produced by epidermal injection or hives

INJECTION INSERTION ANGLES
FOR INTRAMUSCULAR, SUBCUTANEOUS, AND INTRADERMAL SITES

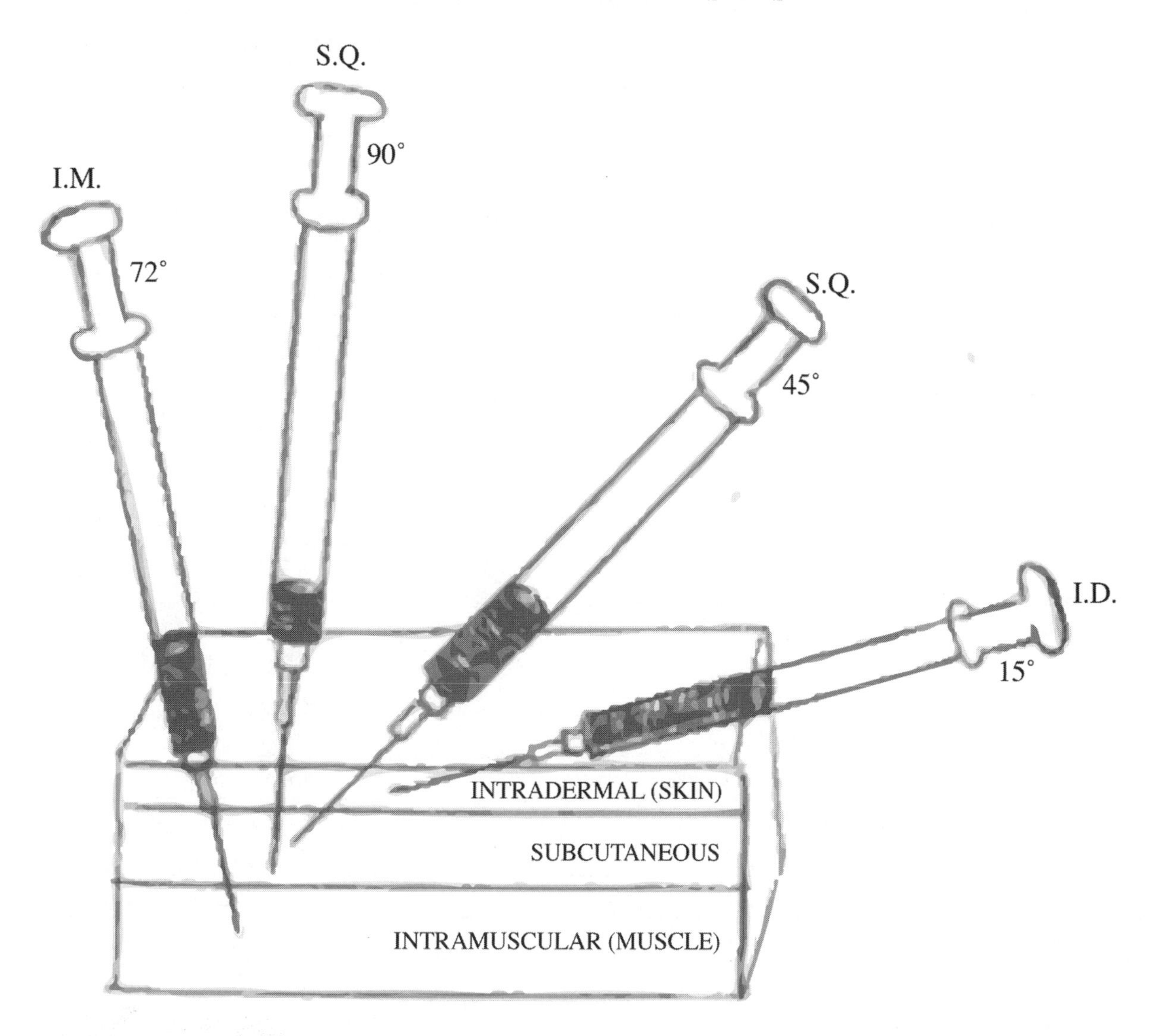

STUDY GUIDE: CONDITIONS OR INJURIES

TERMS	PRONOUNCIATIONS	DEFINITIONS
albinism	(al-bin-izm)	white skin & hair due to lack of pigment
alopecia	(al-o-pes-e-a)	baldness
anaphylactic	(an-a-fil-ak-tik)	severe and potentially fatal allergic response
carcinoma	(kar-sin-o-ma)	cancerous new growth, neoplasm, or tumor
cellulitis	(sel-u-li-tus)	a subcutaneous and connective tissue inflammation (may be fatal)
cicatrix	(sik-a-trix)	scar

TERMS	PRONOUNCIATIONS	DEFINITIONS
contusion	(kon-tu-shun)	black and blue bruise (with no break in skin)
ecchymosis	(ek-ke-mo-sis)	black and blue bruise (due to break in skin)
decubitus	(de-ku-bi-tus)	position of lying down or bedsore/ ulcer on bony prominences from lying for long periods
eczema	(ek-zem-a)	allergic skin redness, often with pruritus (itch)
erythema	(er-ith-e-ma)	redness
exfoliation	(x-fol-e-a-shun)	flaking off of dry skin
exsanquinate	(ex-san-kwin-at)	bleed out
gangrene	(gan-green)	necrotic tissue destruction
hematoma	(he-ma-to-ma)	new growth of blood or bruise due to bleeding under the skin
hidrosis	(hi-dro-sis)	condition of fluid loss or sweating
hirsutism	(hur-sut-izm)	excessive body hair
impetigo	(im-pet-i-go)	communicable pustular lesions caused by staph (treated with antibiotics)
jaundice	(jawn-dus)	yellow-orange colored tissues
keloid	(ke-loyd)	abnormal scar formation
keratosis	(ker-a-to-sis)	thick horn-like skin condition caused by the sun
laceration	(las-er-a-shun)	a cut in the skin, torn tissue
lupus erythematosis	(lu-pus)	butterfly-like skin redness (illness)
mastitis	(mas-ti-tis)	breast inflammation
nevus	(ne-vus)	mole or birthmark (nevi=plural)
nummular	(num-u-lar)	dime sized or shaped
onychitis	(o-nik-i-tus)	nail inflammation
paronychia	(par-o-nik-e-a)	inflammation around a nail
pediculosis	(ped-ik-u-lo-sis)	communicable condition of lice infestation
petechiae	(pet-e-ke-i)	small, flat spontaneous hemorrhagic lesions
pruritus	(prur-i-tus)	itching
psoriasis	(sor-i-as-is)	chronic, hereditary dermatosis with scales
rhytidectomy	(rit-i-dek-to-me)	process of surgical wrinkle excision
scabies	(ska-bez)	communicable mite infestation

TERMS	PRONOUNCIATIONS	DEFINITIONS
steatoma	(ste-a-to-ma)	fatty new growth, neoplasm, or tumor
subungual	(sub-un-kwal)	under the nail
tanorexia	(tan-or-x-e-a)	condition related to excessive use of tanning beds (due to self perception as unacceptably pale despite the known negative side effects - like skin cancer)
tinea	(tin-e-a)	communicable fungus infection (ringworm)
urticaria	(urt-ik-ar-e-a)	hives
verruca	(ver-uk-a)	wart
vitiligo	(vit-il-ag-o)	white patches on skin due to pigment loss

PRACTICE, PRACTICE, PRACTICE...........

Exercise 1:

As soon as you have received new medical terms, begin to review.
Using blank 3"X5" index cards, create flashcards to review all of the new medical terms in this chapter by writing each of the correctly spelled terms five times on one side of the index card and the definition of each term on the other side of the index card. Keeping all of these cards in your right pocket, continually review all of the cards throughout the day. Whenever you have learned a card, place it in your left pocket. After you have learned all of these new terms, periodically refresh your memory with review.

Exercise 2:

Picture this term... what am I? Draw, color, and identify the medical terms for the following described skin lesions and conditions.

Description | Identify The Medical Term | Draw It

1) Bald or a condition called ____________________________

2) Bruise (from bumping into a wall) or ____________________

3) Condition of bruise (after a blood test) or________________

4) Any flat, discolored skin lesion or a____________________

5) A birthmark, mole, or ______________________________

6) A wart or a _______________________________________

7) A large blister (clear fluid filled lesion) or a ______________

8) A raised, discolored skin lesion or a_____________________

9) A skin lesion with bacteria or non-clear fluid: a____________

10) A condition of mite infestation or _____________________

Exercise 3:

Using outside resources, research all medical conditions in this chapter. Write one paragraph of information including a general description, symptoms, and treatment for each of these medical conditions. Be prepared to informally present this written report as part of an in-class review then to hand in your written report next class.

ANSWER KEY: 1) alopecia, 2) contusion, 3) ecchymosis, 4) macule, 5) nevus, 6) verruca, 7) bulla, 8) papule, 9) pustule 10) scabies.

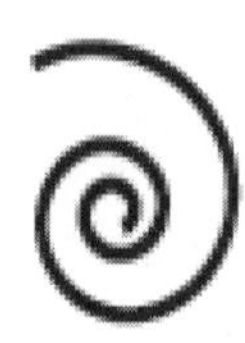

Chapter 11

Musculoskeletal System
The musculoskeletal system functions as a source of physical support as well as protection for the internal organs, as a means of movement, and as a genesis for blood cells.

UPPER AND LOWER EXTREMITIES

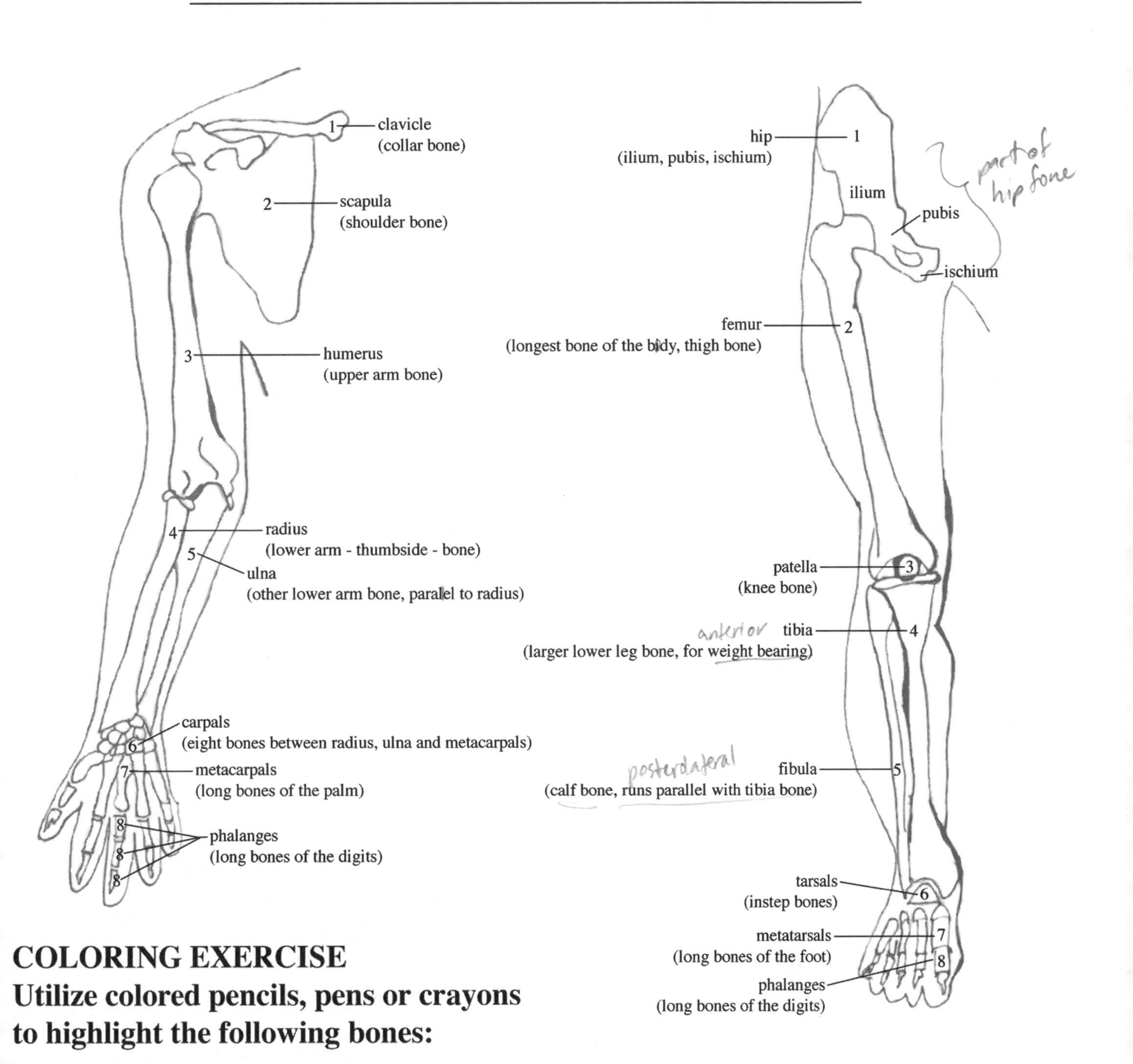

COLORING EXERCISE
Utilize colored pencils, pens or crayons to highlight the following bones:

STUDY GUIDE:

BONE TERMS	PRONOUNCIATIONS	DEFINITIONS
clavicle	(klav-ik-el)	collarbone
scapula	(skap-u-la)	shoulder bone
humerus	(hum-er-us)	upper arm bone
radius	(rad-e-us)	lower arm bone, thumb side
ulna	(ul-na)	lower arm bone, paralell to radius
sternum	(ster-num)	breast bone
vertebral column	~	7 cervical, 12 thoracic, 5 lumbar, 5 sacral, & 4 coccyx: spinal bones
femur	(fe-mur)	thigh bone (longest body bone)
fibula	(fib-u-la)	posterior lower leg bone
tibia	(tib-e-a)	anterior lower leg bone, for weight bearing
mandible	(man-dib-el)	lower jaw bone
patella	(pat-el-a)	knee bone
metacarpals	(meta-kar-pals)	hand bones, long bones of palm
metatarsals	(meta-tar-sals)	foot bones
pelvis	(pel-vis)	pelvic girdle bone
phalanges	(fa-lan-gez)	digits: fingers or toes
amytrophic	(am-i-trof-ik)	related to degenerative development of the motor neurons
anklyosis	(ank-le-o-sis)	condition of joint immobility
arthralgia	(arth-ral-ja)	joint pain
articulation	(ar-tik-u-la-shun)	joint juncture
asthenia	(as-then-e-a)	without strength
ataxia	(a-tax-e-a)	without muscular coordination
atonic	(a-to-ne-a)	without muscular tone
atrophy	(a-tro-fe)	without the process of development (often due to lack of use)
bone marrow	(mar-ro)	the interior filling within a bone cavity (blood cells are produced within red bone marrow)
bursa	(bur-sa)	a fluid filled sac that prevents joint friction
bursitis	(bur-si-tis)	inflammation of the bursa
carpal tunnel syndrome or C.T.S.	(kar-pal tun-nel sin-drom)	inflammation of the median nerve associated with excessive use (sx: carpalgia, edema, numbness, &/or atrophy)
cartilage	(kar-ti-laj)	a type of connective tissue
chondriasis	(kon-dri-a-sis)	condition of cartilage
clonic	(klon-ik)	related to muscular contraction and relaxation
tonic	(ton-ik)	related to muscular tension

BONE TERMS	PRONOUNCIATIONS	DEFINITIONS
contracture	(kon-trak-tur)	muscular contraction
dysynovia	(dis-no-ve-a)	related to difficult or painful synovial fluid
dystrophy	(dis-tro-fe)	difficult or painful development process
fascia	(fas-e-a)	related to fibrous binding for muscle fiber
ganglion	(gang-le-on)	a long bone cyst
gout	(g-out)	a form of acute arthritis that starts with the big toe, foot, or knee (caused by uric and uric salts in the joints)
herniated disk	(H.N.D.)	a ruptured intervertebral disk that has moved into the spinal cord (a slipped disk)
hypertrophy	(hi-per-tro-fe)	excessive development process
hypotrophy	(hi-po-tro-fe)	underdevelopment process
ilium	(il-i-um)	the upper portion of the pelvis
joint	(joynt)	the articulation or junction between two bones
kinesialgia	(kin-es-e-alg-e-a)	pain upon movement
kyphosis	(ki-fo-sis)	condition of hunchback spinal curvature
lateral	(lat-er-al)	side, related to the
ligament	(lig-a-ment)	a portion of connective tissue that joins one bone to another bone
lordosis	(lor-do-sis)	condition of a convex or swayback spinal curvature
luxation	(lux-a-shun)	dislocation
Lyme disease	(lim dis-ez)	a spirochete infection secondary to a deer tick bite (treated with antibiotics)
meniscus	(men-is-cus)	crescent shaped cartilage found within some joints
myelomeningocele	(mi-el-o-men-ing-o-sel)	herniation of the spinal cord and meninges
myelotomy	(mi-el-ot-o-me)	process of incision into the bone marrow
myasthenia gravis	(mi-as-the-ne-a grav-is)	an autoimmune disorder causing muscular paresis and paralysis
nucleus poposus	(nu-kle-us pol-po-sis)	the middle of an intervertebral disk
ossification	(os-if-ik-a-shun)	bone tissue formation
osteoarthritis	(os-te-o-arth-ri-tis)	inflammation of the joint bone
osteomalacia	(os-te-o-mal-a-sha)	a bone softening disease (due to a vitamin D deficiency or renal dysfunction
osteoporosis	(os-te-o-por-o-sis)	condition of bone mass reduction (resulting in porousness of bone, weakness, or fracture)

BONE TERMS	PRONOUNCIATIONS	DEFINITIONS
paralysis	(par-al-is-is)	lack of muscular contraction function
paresis	(par-e-sis)	weakness (remarkable)
hemiparesis	(hem-i-par-e-sis)	half or one-sided weakness
quadriplegia	(kwa-dri-ple-ge-a)	paralysis of all four limbs
rickets	(rik-ets)	a vitamin D and calcium deficiency (can result in developmental deformities for kids)
sarcoma	(sar-ko-ma)	a bone tumor, new growth, or neoplasm
scoliosis	(sko-le-o-sis)	condition of a lateral 'S' spine curvature
spina bifida	(spi-nal bif-i-da)	a congenital spinal defect
spinal stenosis	(spi-nal sten-o-sis)	a condition of spinal canal narrowing (results in pain, pressure, or paresis)
synovial fluid	(sin-ov-e-al flu-id)	the fluid surrounding a joint that promotes free movement
systemic lupus erythematosus or S.L.E.	(sis-tem-ik loo-pus ir-e-them-a-to-sus)	chronic inflammatory disease of connective tissue that causes injury throughout the body (often heralded in by butterfly-shaped facial lesions)
torsion	(tor-shun)	twist, twisting

WRIST AND HAND BONES

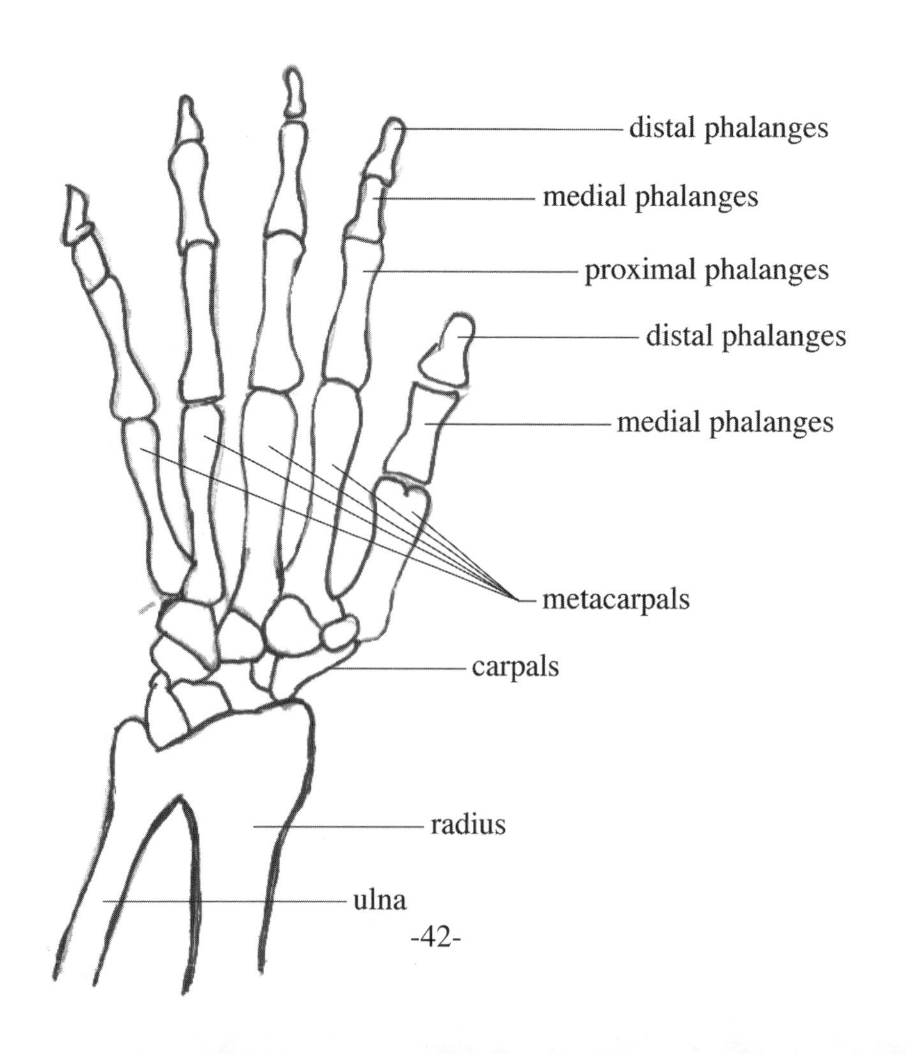

STUDY GUIDE: PROCEDURAL AND TREATMENT

BONE TERMS	PRONOUNCIATIONS	DEFINITIONS
amputation	(am-pu-ta-shun)	partial or complete limb removal
arthrocentesis	(arth-ro-sen-te-sis)	joint puncture to remove fluid
arthroscopy	(arth-ro-skop-e)	procedure or process of joint examination with an instrument
electrical stimulation	(e-lek-trik)	electrical impulses used to heal tendon and cartilage injuries
myelogram	(mi-el-o-gram)	a diagnostic dye-imaging x-ray for the spinal cord
reduction	(re-duk-shun)	spinal fusion
sclerosis	(skler-o-sis)	condition of hardening
spondylosyndesis	(spon-dil-o-sin-de-sis)	spinal fusion
traction	(trak-shun)	related to drawing or pulling procedure

ABBREVIATIONS	DEFINITIONS
A.L.S.	amyotrophic lateral sclerosis
C.T.S.	carpal tunnel syndrome
D.J.D.	degenerative joint disease or osteoarthritis
E.M.G.	electromyography
FX	fracture
H.N.P.	herniated nucleus pulposis
I.M.	intramuscular
L.D.	Lyme disease
L.E.	lupus erythematosis
M.D.	muscular dystrophy
M.G.	myasthenia gravis
N.S.A.I.D.	non-steroidal anti-inflammatory drug
O.T.	occupational therapy
P.T.	physical therapy
R.A.	rheumatoid arthritis
R.I.C.E.	rest, ice, compression, and elevation
R.O.M.	range of motion
S.L.E.	systemic lupus erythematosis

NORMAL VERTEBRAL COLUMNS AND COMMON SPINAL CURVATURES

ANTERIOR VERTEBRAL PERSPECTIVES

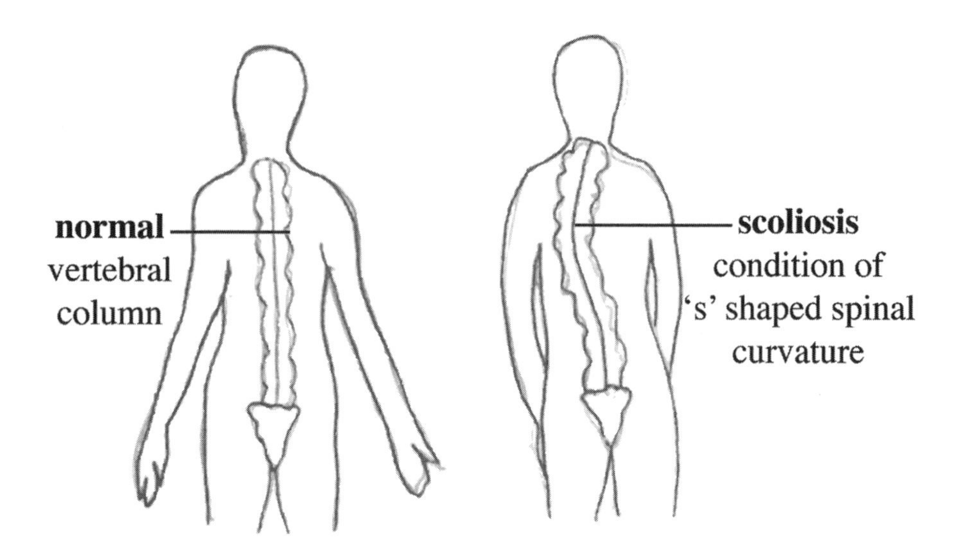

SAGITTAL VERTEBRAL PERSPECTIVES

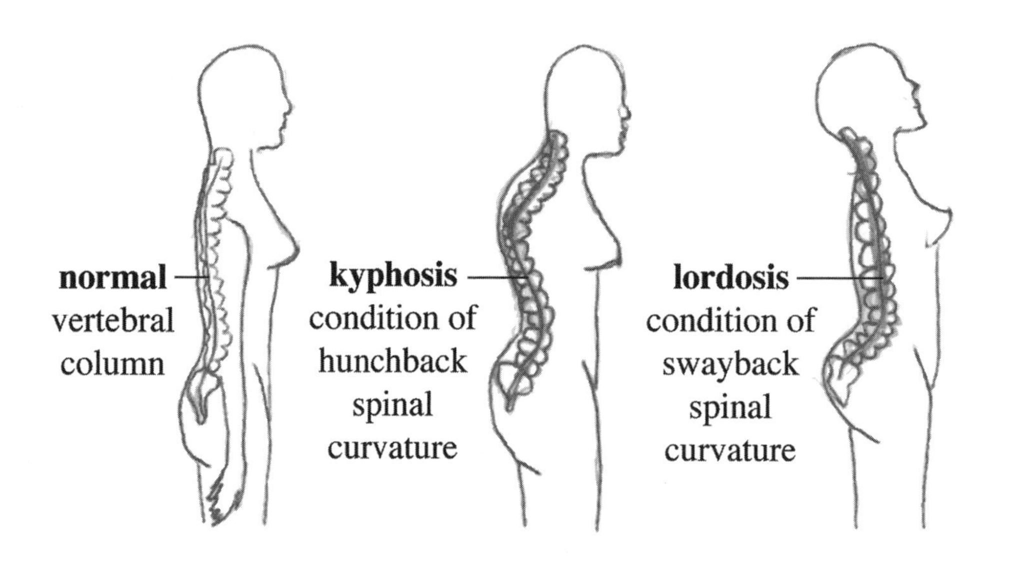

PRACTICE, PRACTICE, PRACTICE..........

Exercise 1:

As soon as you have received new medical terms, begin to review. Using blank 3"X5" index cards, create flashcards to review all of the new medical terms in this chapter by writing each of the correctly spelled terms five times on one side of the index card and the definition of each term on the other side of the index card.

Keeping all of these cards in your right pocket, continually review all of the cards throughout the day. Whenever you have learned a card, place it in your left pocket. After you have learned all of these new terms, periodically refresh your memory with review.

Exercise 2:
With or without a study buddy; create a poem, a song, or a three dimensional object that will help you as well as your class remember any ten medical terms from this chapter.

Exercise 3:
Whereabout Scout. Utilize colored pencils, pens, and/ or crayons to color as well as identify bones of the upper and lower extremities.

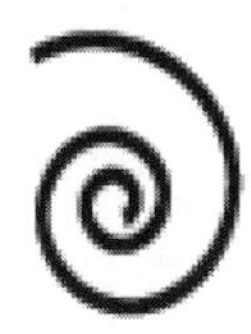

Chapter 12

Cardiovascular System
The cardiovascular system maintains circulation by sending nutrients and oxygen t
body cells as well as taking carbon dioxide and toxins to the lungs for elimination.

THE HEART

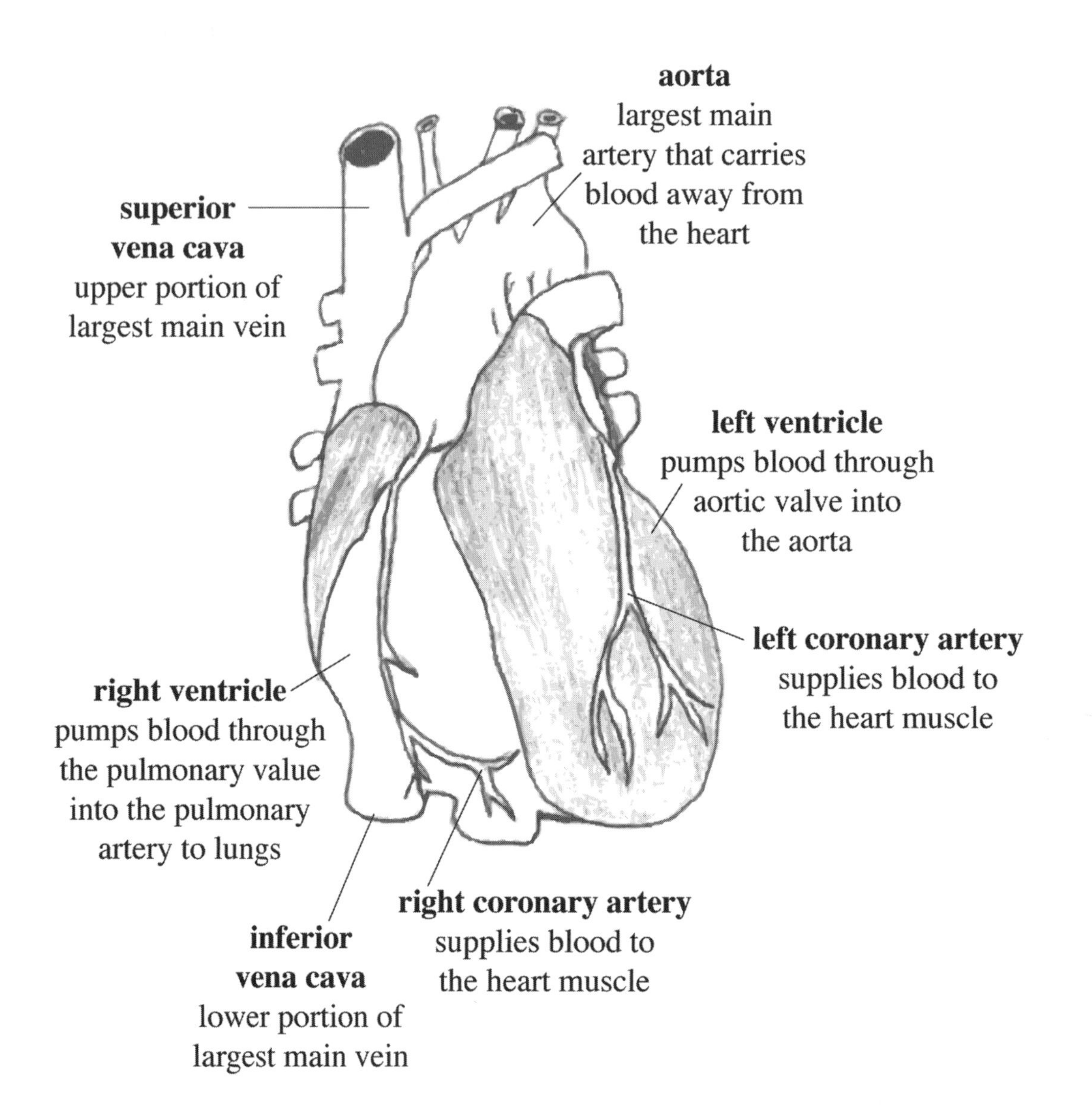

STUDY GUIDE: ANATOMICAL

TERMS	PRONOUNCIATIONS	DEFINITIONS
aorta	(a-or-ta)	largest / main artery
arteries	(art-er-ez)	vessels that carry oxygenated blood away from the heart
capillaries	(kap-il-ar-ez)	small vessels connecting arteries and veins

TERMS	PRONOUNCIATIONS	DEFINITIONS
oronary arteries	(kor-on-ar-e)	vessels that supply blood to the heart muscle
inoatrial node	(si-no-a-tre-al nod)	the pacemaker
eins	(vanz)	vessels carry de-O_2 blood to the heart
alves	(valvs)	keeps blood from flowing backwards
ena cava	(ve-na ka-va)	largest/ main vein
iastolic	(di-as-tol-ik)	related to the ventricular relaxation phase of the heart cycle
ystolic	(sis-tol-ik)	related to the ventricular contraction within the heart cycle
ypertension	(hi-perpten-shun)	high blood pressure
ypotension	(hi-po-ten-swhun)	low blood pressure
tenosis	(sten-o-sis)	condition of narrowing
estenosis	(restenosis)	return to the condition of narrowing
mbolus	(em-bo-lus)	a free-floating clot of air, blood, fat, bacteria, or foreign body that could lodge
hrombus	(throm-bus)	a stationary blood clot
radycardia	(bra-de-kar-de-a)	slow heart rate
achycardia	(tak-e-kar-de-a)	fast heart rate

TUDY GUIDE:

TERMS	PRONOUNCIATIONS	DEFINITIONS
neurysm	(an-yur-izm)	a weak and ballooned vessel wall
ngina pectoris	(an-ji-na pek-tor-is)	chest pain
ngioplasty	(an-ge-o-plas-te)	process or procedure of reconstructing the a blood vessel canal to open the lumen
rrhythmia	(a-rith-me-a)	related to without rhythm
therosclerosis	(ath-er-o-skler-o-sis)	condition of fatty plaque deposits hardening and narrowing arterial walls
trial fibrillation	(a-tre-al fib-ril-a-shun)	irregular heartbeat occuring in two upper chambers that causes an absence of p-waves
ardiac arrest	(kar-de-ak ar-rest)	a complete cessation of electrical and/ or mechanical cardiac activity
ardiac catheterization	(kar-de-ak kath)	intracardiac arterial tube insertion to measure pressures and evaluate function of the heart
ardiopulmonary resuscitation or CPR	(kar-de-o pulm-on-ar-e re-sus-si-ta-shun)	an emergency procedure aimed at restoring ventilation and cardiac functions
ardioversion	(kar-de-o-ver-shun)	return to normal heartbeat
-reactive protein	(c-re-ak-tiv)	a blood test that assesses risk of heart attack (over 3mg./liter)
yanosis	(si-an-o-sis)	condition of blueness

TERMS	PRONOUNCIATIONS	DEFINITIONS
diaphoresis	(di-a-for-e-sis)	profuse perspiration
dysequilibrium	~	generalized sensation of unsteadiness generally related to hypotension, hypertension, hyperventilation or poor circulation
electrocardiogram	(ECG or EKG)	a graphic recording of cardiac activity
extrasystole	(x-tra-sis-to-le)	premature heart contraction
fibrillation	(fi-bril-a-shun)	fast but incomplete heartbeat
head up tilt testing	(HUTT)	continual B/P and E.C.G. monitoring on a tilting (to 60 degrees) table for 45 minutes
hypercholestemia	(hi-per-ko-les-tem-e-a)	excessive/ high blood cholesterol
intracardiac catheterization or ccath	(in-tra kar-de-ak)	cardiac catheterization
ischemia	(is-kem-e-a)	insufficient blood/ O2 to a tissue
infarct	(in-farkt)	an obstruction
intermittent claudification or I.T.C.	(in-ter-mit-ent klaw-dif-ik-a-shun)	muscular movement pain (due to a poor blood supply)
blood pressure	(B/P)	the pressure or force exerted on vessel walls by blood circulation. B/P is measured in a systolic/ diastolic ratio expressed in millimeters of mercury (mm)
systolic	(sis-tol-ik)	the upper number of a blood pressure reading that represents the greatest force of blood from ventricular contraction on a vessel wall (normal=120mmHg or lower)
diastolic	(di-a-stol-ik)	the lower number of a blood pressure reading that represents the least force of blood from ventricular relaxation on a vessel wall (normal=80mmHg or lower)
hypotension	(hi-po-ten-shun)	low blood pressure
hypertension	(hi-per-ten-shun)	high blood pressure: - systolic of 140 mmHg or higher - diastolic of 90 mmHg or higher
tamponade	(tam-po-nad)	compression created by fluid accumulation in the pericardial sac (may cause coronary vessel issue)

****

Know the 411:

According to The National Institutes of Health:

- 38% of women will die within one year after having a heart attack.
- While 1 in 30 U.S. women die of breast cancer, 1 in 2 U.S. women die of heart disease or stroke.

Classic M.I.: One or more of the following sx noted mainly in males: (denial)

- squeezing angina or chest pressure/fullness/tightness (lasting more than a few minutes, goes away then returns)
- S.O.B. (shortness of breath)
- diaphoresis (excessive perspiration)

numbnesss, tingling or radiating discomfort in arm, jaw, neck, shoulder, back, or stomach
abdominal issues (such as dyspepsia, heartburn, indigestion and/or belching)
nausea or malaise
pallor
syncope or sudden vertigo
fatigue/unexplained exhaustion

According to The Cleveland Heart and Vascular Institute, women tend to have the following heart attack sx 10 years later than men:
exhaustion
S.O.B. (shortness of breath)
paresis (weakness)
diaphoresis (cold sweat/excessive persipiration)
jaw pain
feeling anxious or as if something is wrong

****

BALLOON ANGIOPLASTY

sheath - a tube used to facilitate and deploy stent placement

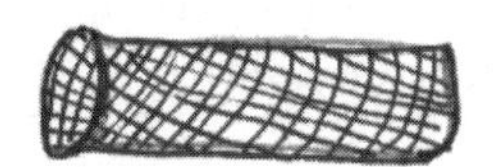

stent - a cylindric shaped hollow rod (often composed of wire mesh the diameter approximately of a ballpoint pen's ink cartridge) that is used to assure patency of a lumen.

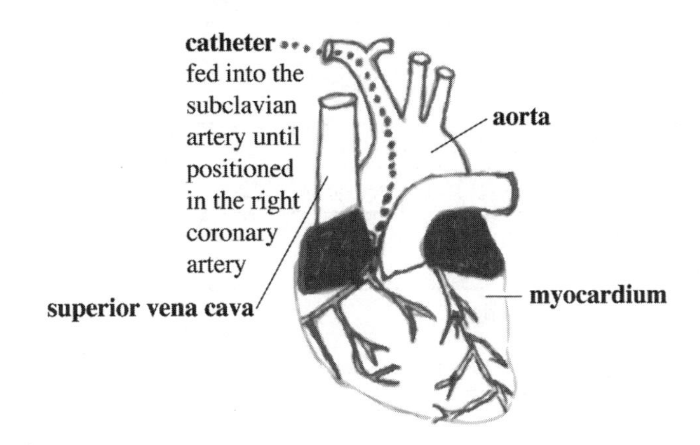

A catheter is gently threaded into the subclavian artery then an angiogram locates the precise location of plague blockage. The balloon catheter is inflated within the blocked vessel to open the passageway. After the catheter is removed, a stent may or may not be inserted to assist in maintaining vessel patency (openess). (Any remaining plaque is generally broken down and eliminated).

1 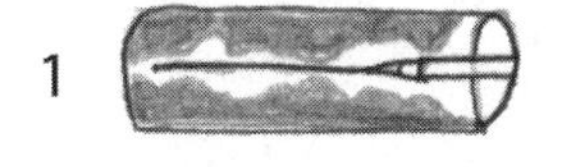 introduction: tip of the catheter enters coronary vessel blocked with plaque

2 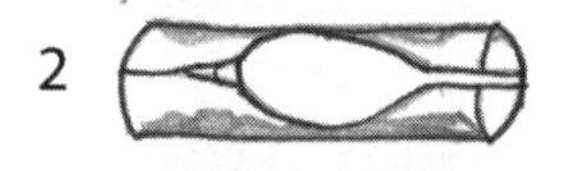 catheter inflation

3 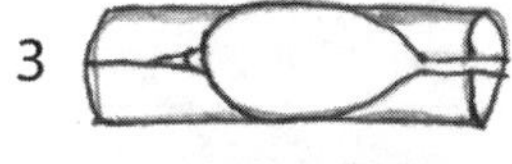 plaque compression and lumen patent

4 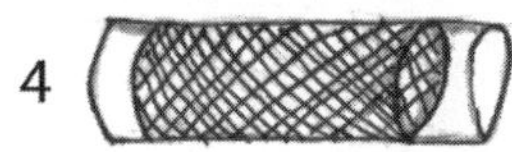 stent in place to maintain lumen patency

****

Know the 911:

myocardial infarction (mi-o-kar-de-al in-farkt) or M.I.	coronary artery blockage (heart attack) that leads to heart muscle tissue death. Sx may include: - denial - flu-like sx:nausea,malaise - vertigo - unexplained exhaustion - pallor - angina pectoris lasting more than a few minutes, goes away then returns - SOB - diaphoresis - uncomfortable chest pressure, fullness, or squeezing - radiating discomfort to jaw, arm, back, or stomach - abdominal issues (indigestion, belching, fullness, or burning sensation)
cardiac arrest	a complete cessation of electrical and/ or mechanical cardiac activity characterized by a sudden loss of responsiveness, no normal breathing, no pulse, no coughing, and/ or no movement.

If one or more of these symptoms emerge, IMMEDIATELY CALL 9-1-1.
Questions? Call the American Heart Association 1-800-242-8721
or see http://www.americanheart.org/

****

STUDY GUIDE: TERMS AND ABBREVIATIONS

TERMS	PRONOUNCIATIONS	DEFINITIONS
metabolic syndrome or M.B.S. or syndrome x	(met-a-bol-ik sindrom)	confluence of obesity, hypertension, diabetes, then heart disease
Moyamoya disease	(moy-a-moy-a)	a disease of intravascular stenosis and ischemic events
occlusion	(o-klu-shun)	blockage or obstruction
pallor	(pal-or)	pale or paleness
perfusion	(per-fu-shun)	passage of fluid through an organ or tissue
rheumatic heart disease	(ru-mat-ik)	strep infection damaging heart valves
sinus rhythm	(si-nus ri-thum)	normal heart rhythm
syncope	(sin-ko-pe)	faint or temporary loss of consciousness
syndrome x or metabolic syndrome	(sin-drom x)	metabolic syndrome
transtelephonic monitoring	(TPM)	monitor wearing that records electrical impulses that store ECG recordings that are transmitted via telephone

ABBREVIATIONS	DEFINITIONS
A	airway maintenance
B	breathing

ABBREVIATIONS	DEFINITIONS
C	circulation
D	disability
E	exposure
ABP	arterial blood pressure
ACLS	advanced cardiac life support
AF, afib, or atfib	atrial fibrillation
AMI	acute myocardial infarction
ASCVD	arteriosclerotic cardiovascular disease
ASHD	arteriosclerotic heart disease
BP or B/P	blood pressure
CA	cardiac arrest, cardiac arrhythmia, or cancer
CABG	coronary artery bypass graft
CABS	coronary artery bypass surgery
CAD	coronary artery disease
CCU	Coronary Care Unit
CEA	carotid endarterectomy
CHD	coronary heart disease
CHF	congestive heart failure
CPR	cardiopulmonary resuscitation
CRP	c-reactive protein
CRT	cardiac resynchronization therapy
GT	glucose test
DNR	do not resuscitate
DVT	deep vein thrombosis
ECHO	echocardiogram
ECG	electrocardiogram
EKG	electrocardiogram
ETT	exercise tolerance test or treadmill stress test
EVAR	endovascular aneurysm repair
HDL	high density lipoproteins
HTN	hypertension
HUTT	head-up tilt table
ICD	implantable cardioverter defibrillator
IVC	intraventricular catheter
LDL	low density lipoproteins
LVH	left ventricular hypertrophy
MI	myocardial infarction (heart attack)
MS	mitral stenosis
MVP	mitral valve prolapse
NAK	sodium potassium
NSR	normal sinus rhythm
O2	oxygen

ABBREVIATIONS	DEFINITIONS
P	pulse
PAD	peripheral artery disease
PCI	percutaneous coronary intervention (stent)
PDA	patent ductus arteriosis
PIC	peripheral intravenous catheter
PTCA	percutaneous transluminal coronary angioplasty
PVC	premature ventricular contraction
RHD	rheumatic heart disease
SA	sinoatrial
SVT	supraventricular tachycardia
TET	treadmill exercise test
TIA	transient ischemic attack (mini-stroke)
TPM	transtelephonic monitoring
VF	ventricular fibrillation
VLDL	very low density lipoprotein
v-tach	ventricular tachycardia

PRACTICE, PRACTICE, PRACTICE...........

Exercise 1:

As soon as you have received new medical terms, begin to review. Using blank 3"X5" index cards, create flashcards to review all of the new medical terms in this chapter by writing each of the correctly spelled terms five times on one side of the index card and the definition of each term on the other side of the index card. Keeping all of these cards in your right pocket, continually review all of the cards throughout the day. Whenever you have learned a card, place it in your left pocket. After you have learned all of these new terms, periodically refresh your memory with review.

Exercise 2:

Build a Word. Given the definition, build the medical term it represents.

Definition — Medical Term

1) The condition of narrowing = ______________________________

2) Related to a fast heart (rate) = ______________________________

3) The process or procedure of vessel reconstruction = ______________________________

4) The condition of blueness = ______________________________

5) Vein inflammation = ______________________________

6) The condition of having stationary blood clots = ______________________________

7) A weakened, ballooned portion of vessel = ______________________________

8) High blood pressure = ______________________________

9) Faint or temporary loss of consciousness = ______________________________

10) Related to insufficient blood/ O2 to a tissue = ______________________________

11) The condition of arterial hardening = ______________________________

12) Chest pain = ______________________________

13) Related to ventricular contraction = ______________________________

14) Any disease process of the heart muscle = ______________________________

15) Profuse perspiration = ______________________________

- Research the abnormal heart sounds: bruit and gallop then share the information in class.

Exercise 3:

Promote a Heart Tour. Design a tourist guide for the heart. Explain the anatomical highlights and sell the merit of their contributions to bodily function. (Ask your instructor if you may earn extra-credit for color design, outside professional reference utilization, or special features your brochure may offer). Be prepared to share your brochure with the class.

ANSWER KEY: 1) stenosis, 2) tachycardia, 3) angioplasty, 4) cyanosis, 5) phlebitis, 6) thrombosis, 7) aneurysm, 8) hypertension, 9) syncope, 10) ischemia, 11) arteriosclerosis, 12) angina pectoris, 13) systolic, 14) cardiomyopathy, and 15) diaphoresis.

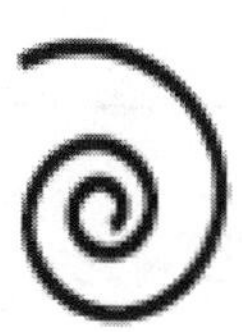

Chapter 13

Respiratory System
The respiratory system sends oxygen to bodily tissues and removes carbon dioxide.

STUDY GUIDE: ANATOMICAL

TERMS	PRONOUNCIATIONS	DEFINITIONS
pharynx	(far-anx)	throat
larynx	(lar-anx)	voice box
trachea	(tra-ke-a)	windpipe
bronchi	(bron-ki)	the two main tracheal branches
bronchioles	(bron-ki-ols)	the smaller branches of the bronchus
alveoli	(al-ve-o-li)	the small air sacs wherein gas is exchanged
diaphragm	(di-a-fram)	the dome-shaped muscle powering respiration
eustachian tube	(u-sta-shun)	tube that equalizes pharyngeal/middle ear pressure
epiglottis	(ep-i-glo-is)	a tracheal flap (that usually closes when swallowing)
pleura	(pler-a)	insulating mucous membrane that covers the lung
tonsils	(ton-sils)	filtering tissue in back of the throat
adenoids	(ad-en-oyds)	filtering tissue in back of the nose
uvula	(u-vu-la)	a dangling muscle tissue that protects the nasal opening on the soft palate
allergen	(al-er-jen)	any environmental agent that causes an allergic reaction
anoxia	(an-ox-e-a)	related to without oxygen
aphonia	(a-fo-ne-a)	without voice (related to a laryngeal issue)
apnea	(ap-ne-a)	without breathing
asphyxiation	(as-fix-e-a-shun)	breathing suffocation
aspiration	(as-pir-a-shun)	choke, breath in stomach contents, or withdraw fluid
asthma	(az-ma)	a chronic, obstructive, lung disease with sx of wheezing
atelectasis	(at-el-ek-tas-is)	collapsed lung due to trauma or obstruction
auscultation	(as-kul-ta-shun)	listening to sounds (breath, bowel, or heart)
breath sound	(breth-so-und)	audible sounds during respiration (rales, rhonchi, stridor, or wheeze)
bronchoconstriction or B.C.N.	(bron-ko-kon-strik-shun)	a small lung airway narrowing due to muscular tightening

TERMS	PRONOUNCIATIONS	DEFINITIONS
Cheyne-Stokes	(chan-soks)	a cycle of irregular breathing (shallow and slow then deeper and faster to slow with 10-20 second periods of stopping followed by repetition of this sequencing)
chronic obstructive pulmonary disease	(kron-ik ab-struk-tiv)	irreversably decreased lung function
coryza	(kor-i-za)	a common virus, a cold
croup	(krup)	an acute pediatric condition with stridor and a barking cough
cyanosis	(si-an-o-sis)	a condition of blueness (due to insufficient O2 to tissues)
dysphonia	(dis-fo-ne-a)	difficult or painful voice (related to laryngeal issues)
dyspnea	(disp-ne-a)	difficult or painful breathing
effusion	(ef-u-shun)	a flowing out of fluid or gas
emphysema	(em-fi-se-ma)	an irreversible chronic pulmonary disease (distended alveoli)
epistaxis	(ep-is-tax-is)	a nosebleed
expectoration	(x-pek-tor-a-shun)	lung production or substance that was coughed up
hemoptysis	(he-mop-ti-sis)	blood in expectoration or lung production
hemothorax	(he-mo-thor-ax)	blood in chest cavity
hiatal hernia	(hi-a-tal her-ne-a)	rupture or swelling of the diaphragm
hypercapnea	(hi-per-kap-ne-a)	excessive breathing (and increased blood CO2)
hypoxia	(hi-pox-e-a)	related to low oxygen intake
Legionnaire's disease	(le-jon-ars)	a severe bacillic pneumonia (often with GI issues)
mesothelioma	(me-so-thel-e-o-ma)	a malignant new growth, tumor, or neoplasm of the pleural membrane (often due to asbestos inhalation)
olfaction	(ol-fak-shun)	pertaining to smelling or smell
orthopnea	(or-thop-ne-a)	upright breathing (easier to breathe when sitting up)
patent	(pay-tent)	open or unblocked (for example: a patient's airway or lumen)
pertussis	(per-tus-is)	an acute, communicable bacterial infection (also called "whooping cough")
pleurisy	(pler-is-e)	pleural inflammation with fluid drainage (sx: severe pain, dyspnea, or presence of air/ gas in the pleural cavity)
pneumonia	(nu-mo-ne-a)	related to lung inflammation caused by bacteria, virus, environmental irritants, or fungi

TERMS	PRONOUNCIATIONS	DEFINITIONS
pneumothorax	(new-mo-thor-ax)	air collecting within the chest cavity (causes dyspnea)
pulmonary edema or P.E.	(pulm-on-ar-e ed-em-a)	air/ gas collection in the pleural cavity (may lead to fluid retention in lung)
rales	(ral)	bubbling and rattling breath sounds heard upon auscultation
rhonchi	(ron-ki)	rattling sound heard in the bronchial tubes or throat
respiratory distress syndrome or R.D.S.	(res-pir-a-tor-e dist-tres sin-drom)	lack of lung development (premature infants)
respiratory syncytial virus or R.S.V.	(res-pira-tor-e sin-si-chal- vi-rus)	a communicable URI in infants and children
rhinoplasty	(ri-no-plas-te)	the procedure or process of surgical nose reconstruction
severe acute respiratory syndrome (SARS)	(sev-er a-kut)	a communicable, serious pneumonia
sputum	(spu-tum)	a lung production or a substance that is coughed up
streptococcal pharyngitis	(strep throat)	a communicable bacterial throat infection
stridor	(stri-dor)	an urgent high pitched throat or breath sound
sudden infant death syndrome or S.I.D.S.	~	unexplained death of a seemingly healthy infant
tachypnea	(tak-pne-a)	fast breathing
tuberculosis	(tu-ber-ku-lo-sis)	a communicable bacterial infection with potentially serious systemic reprocussions
wheeze	(wez)	a whistling breath sound
adenoidectomy	(ad-noyd-ek-tom-e)	procedure of surgical excision of the adenoids
Heimlich maneuver	(him-lik)	an emergency technique using diaphragm pressure to remove a foreign body from the trachea, pharynx, or esophagus
hyperbaric oxygen therapy or HBOT	~	oxygen treatment used under greater than normal atmospheric pressure
inhaler	(in-hal-er)	see 'metered dose inhaler'
intermittent positive pressure breathing or IPPB	~	using increased mehanical pressure and mask to assist breathing
intubate	(in-tu-bat)	insertion of a tube (to establish an airway, for an example)
mechanical ventilation	~	an advanced life support method that controls breathing
metered dose inhaler or MDI	~	a portable pressurized device that directs medications to the lungs
nebulizer	(neb-u-li-zer)	a device used to deploy pulmonary medication

TERMS	PRONOUNCIATIONS	DEFINITIONS
postural drainage or PD	~	positioning the chest using gravity to enhance bronchial drainage
pulmonary function test	(PFT)	examination to measure lung volume and gas exchange (in order to determine lung volume)
pulse oximetry	(puls ox-im-e-tre)	procedure or process of measuring the saturation of hemoglobin RBC with oxygen via infared light (95% or greater is normal)
respirator	(res-pir-a-tor)	machine used for long term artificial respiration
spirometry	(spir-om-e-tre)	procedure or process of measuring the pulmonary breathing capacity
suctioning	(suk-shun-ing)	removing secretions by applying negative pressure directly
tonsillectomy	(ton-sil-ek-to-me)	procedure or process of surgical excision of the tonsils
tracheostomy	(tra-ke-os-to-me)	procedure or process of artificially establishing a mouthlike opening into the trachea

THE RESPIRATORY SYSTEM

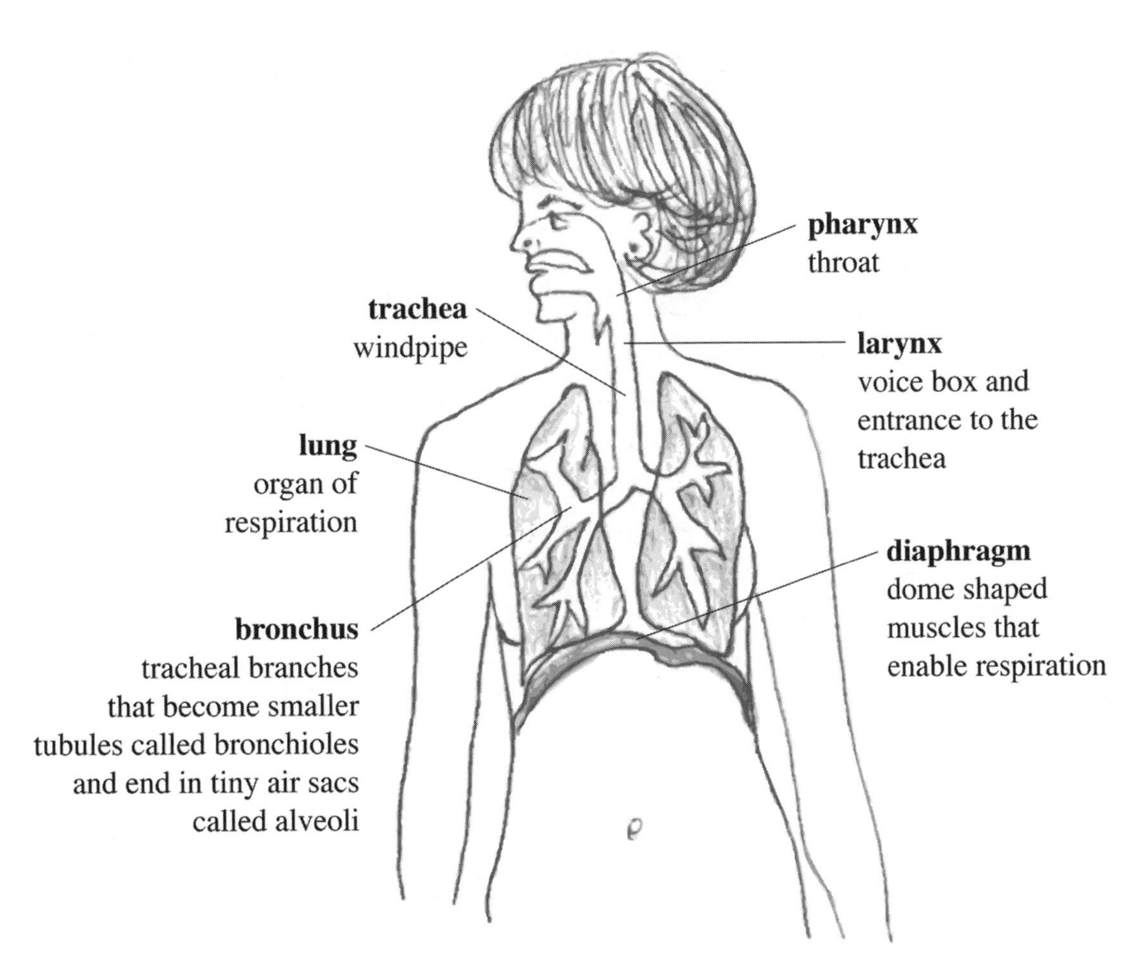

ABBREVIATIONS	DEFINITIONS
A&P	auscultation and percussion
ABG	arterial blood gases
AED	automated external defibrillator
BCG	or Bacille Calmette-Guerin, TB vaccine (not generally recommended unless high risk of TB to prevent childhood tuberculous meningitis and miliary disease)
B2-AGONIST	selective stimulator of B2-adrenergic receptor that relieves airway constriction
BS	breathing sounds
CF	cystic fibrosis
CO2	carbon dioxide
COLD	chronic obstructive lung disease
COPD	chronic obstructive pulmonary disease
CPAP	continuous positive airway pressure
CPE	chronic pulmonary emphysema
CPR	cardiopulmonary resuscitation
CXR	chest x-ray
DPT	diptheria, pertussis, and tetanus (immunization)
ENT	ear, nose, and throat
ET	endotracheal
ETT	endotracheal tube
HBOT	hyperbaric oxygen therapy
IPPB	intermittent positive pressure breathing
LLL	left lower lobe
LUL	left upper lobe
MDI	metered dose inhaler
MDR-TB	multi drug resistant tuberculosis
MRSA	methicillin resistant staphlococcus Aureus infection
O2	oxygen
PFT	pulmonary function test
PO	per os or by mouth
PTX, Pnx, or Px	pneumothorax
R	respiration, rectal or rectally
RDS	respiratory distress syndrome
RLL	right lower lobe
RR	respiratory rate
RSV	respiratory syncytial virus
RUL	right upper lobe
SARS	severe acute respiratory syndrome
SIDS	sudden infant death syndrome
SOB	shortness of breath
T&A	tonsillectomy and adenoidectomy

ABBREVIATIONS	DEFINITIONS
TB	tuberculosis
TCDB	turn, cough, and deep breathe
TLC	total lung capacity or tender loving care
TPR	temperature, pulse, and respiration
URI	upper respiratory infection
VC	vital capacity
XDR-TB	extremely drug resistant tuberculosis

PRACTICE, PRACTICE, PRACTICE...........

Exercise 1:

As soon as you have received new medical terms, begin to review. Using blank 3îX5î index cards, create flashcards to review all of the new medical terms in this chapter by writing each of the correctly spelled terms five times on one side of the index card and the definition of each term on the other side of the index card. Keeping all of these cards in your right pocket, continually review all of the cards throughout the day. Whenever you have learned a card, place it in your left pocket. After you have learned all of these new terms, periodically refresh your memory with review.

Exercise 2:

Spell Check. Correctly spell any medical terms that seem misspelled. Do not refer to the chapter. Check the answer key at the bottom of the next page for the correct spelling of any terms requiring correction. If you encounter any spelling issues after you check your answers, rewrite the correctly spelled medical terms ten times.

Medical Term Correction (?)

1) tonsilectomy ________________
2) epiglottus________________
3) uvala________________
4) anoxea ________________
5) asfixeation ________________

Medical Term Correction (?)

6) koriza ________________
7) epitaxis ________________
8) hemoptisis ________________
9) sputim ________________
10) tachpnea ________________

Exercise 3:

Batting a Thousand. Here's the pitch: go to first base and collect 25 points with a prefix, proceed to second base and collect 25 points for picking up a root word part to add to the prefix, and then collect 25 more points when you pass third base and add a suffix to make a home run of one medical term for a total of 100 points. The object of the game is the creation of ten medical terms/ home runs (which equals 1,000 points). The same prefixes, roots, and suffixes may be used more than once.

Second Base:
Root Word
Parts

ox
tub
hal
optys
pne
phon
metr

Third
Base:
Suffixes

-y
-ia
-a
-is
-ate
-er

First
Base:
Prefixes

a-
spiro-
tachy-
dys-
hypo-
oxi-
in-
hem-

HOME RUNS:
Medical Terms

1)____________________

2)____________________

3)____________________

4)____________________

5)____________________

6)____________________

7)____________________

8)____________________

9)____________________

10)____________________

ANSWER KEY: Exercise 2: 1) tonsillectomy, 2) epiglottis, 3) uvula, 4) anoxia, 5) asphyxiation, 6) coryza, 7) epistaxis, 8) hemoptysis, 9) sputum, 10) tachypnea

Exercise 3: hypoxia, intubate, anoxia, aphonia, inhaler, oximetry, tachypnea, hemoptysis, dysphonia, spirometry

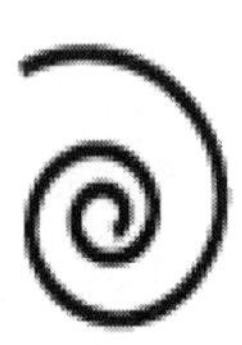

Chapter 14

Gastrointestinal System
The gastrointestinal system or digestive system functions to ingest, digest, and absorb nutrients.

STUDY GUIDE: ANATOMICAL

TERMS	PRONOUNCIATIONS	DEFINITIONS
alimentary canal	(al-im-en-tar-e)	all of the gastrointestinal organs
os	(os)	mouth (or mouthlike opening)
pharynx	(fa-rinx)	throat
esophagus	(e-sof-a-gus)	a tube from the pharynx to the stomach
stomach	(stom-ak)	the muscular sac between the esophagus and duodenum
duodenum	(du-od-en-um)	first of three parts of the small intestine
jejunum	(jej-un-um)	second of three parts of the small intestine
ileum	(il-e-um)	third of three parts of the small intestine
cecum	(se-kum)	sac-like tissue forming the start of the large intestine
appendix	(ap-en-dix)	tissue attached to the cecum
ascending colon	(as-en-ding)	first of four parts of the large intestine
transverse colon	(tranz-vers)	second of four parts of the large intestine
descending colon	(de-send-ing)	third of four parts of the large intestines
sigmoid colon	(sig-moyd)	fourth of four parts of the large intestine
rectum	(rek-tom)	site of waste evacuation from the large intestine
anus	(an-us)	purse string-like muscle sphincter that controls fecal flow
pancreas	(pan-kre-as)	gland that produces digestive enzymes and secretes glucagon as well as insulin
liver	(liv-er)	gland that stores carbohydrates, proteins, and fats (assists with metabolism)
gallbladder	(gal-blad-er)	sac attached to liver that stores extra bile
adhesions	(ad-ha-shuns)	fibrous bands of scar tissue that can displace surrounding organs
anorexia	(an-or-x-e-a-)	without appetite

THE GASTROINTESTINAL OR G.I. SYSTEM

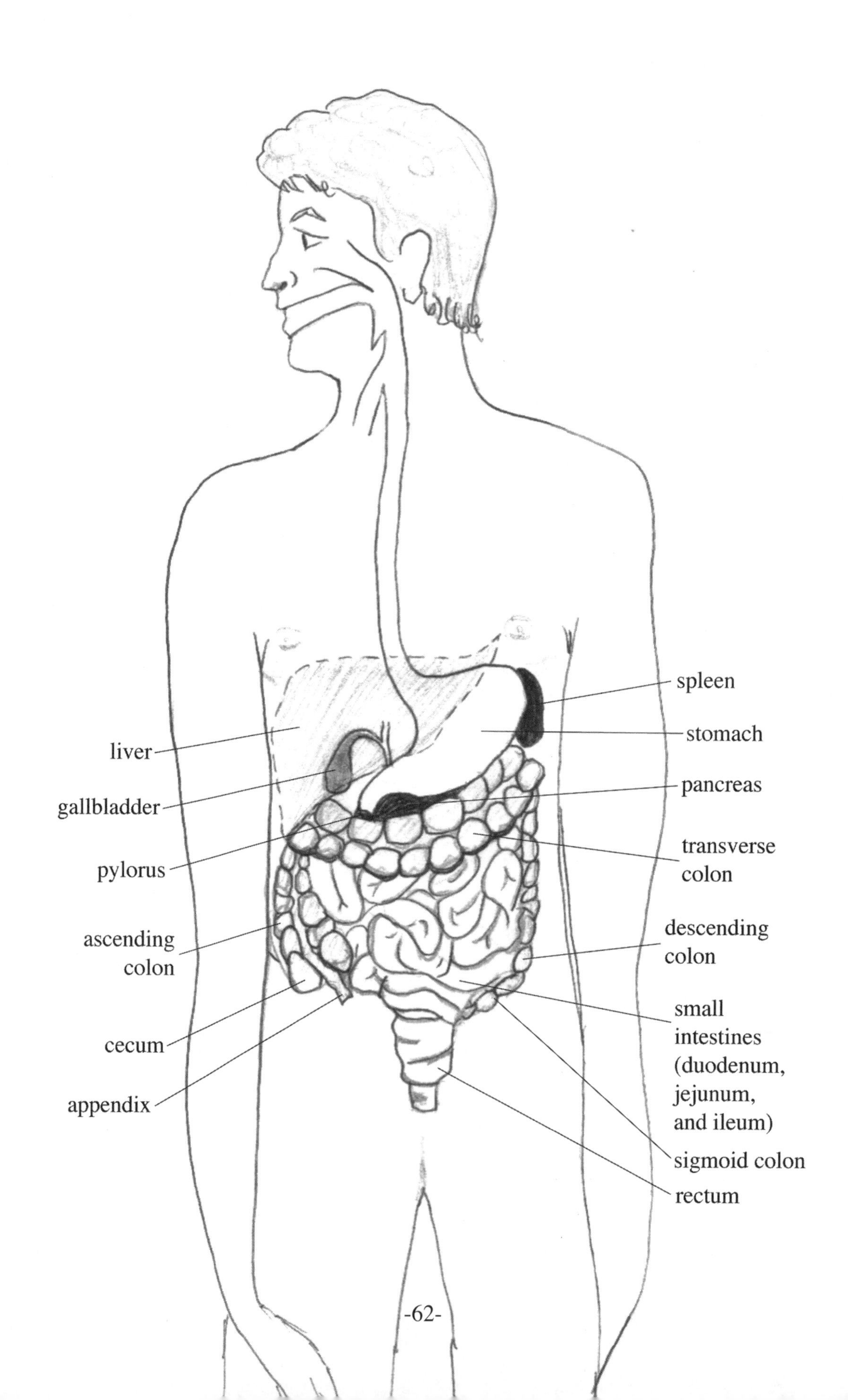

TERMS	PRONOUNCIATIONS	DEFINITIONS
norexia nervosa	(an-or-x-e-a ner-vo-sa)	an eating disorder characterized by a distorted body image, compulsive control, food aversion, fear of weight gain, and layering of clothing (higher death rate than other psychiatric eating issues)
scites	(as-i- tes)	a collection of peritoneal fluid
abesiosis	(bab-es-e-o-sis)	a condition of tick bite infection (with sx of fever, malaise, fatigue, stiff neck, and headache then neurological as well as cardiac issues)
inge eating disorder or B.E.D.	(binj)	eating in excess of 2500 calories within 2 hours with feelings of shame, distress, and physical discomfort at least biweekly for 6 months (beyond hunger, eating to cope with stress)
orborygmi	(bor-bor-ig-mi)	digestive noise or growl
ulimia nervosa	(bul- e-me-a)	an eating disorder involving chronic secretive uncontrolled bingeing during brief amount of time followed by self induced purging with substance abuse, gag reflex stimulation, and/or intense exercise for at least 2 weeks over a 3 week period
holelithiasis	(kol-e-li-thi-a-sis)	a condition of gallbladder stones
irrhosis	(sir-o-sis)	a condition of chronic liver disease
Crohn's disease	(kronz)	a chronically inflamed bowel
istention	(dis-ten-shun)	stretching beyond the normal circumference from internal pressure
iverticulitis	(di-ver-tik-u-li-tis)	inflammation of esophageal or intestinal pouches
iverticulosis	(di-ver-tik-u-lo-sis)	condition of esophogeal or intestinal pouches
yspepsia	(dis-pep-se-a)	difficult or painful digestion
ysphagia	(dis-faj-e-a)	difficult or painful eating or swallowing

otential Medical Complications of Eating Disorders

death
depression
low self esteem
vertigo
cardiac arrhythmia
osteoporesis
reflux
tooth loss
pharyngitis
gastric tear or rupture
hair loss
sluggish intestinal activity
dehydration

- listlessness
- anxiety disorders
- dysphoria
- shortness of breath
- potassium deficiency
- fractures
- amenorrhea
- tooth enamel erosion
- indigestion
- metabolic issues
- cold intolerance
- chronic constipation
- toxicity

- obsessive compulsive disorder
- substance abuse
- hypotension
- chest discomfort
- electrolyte imbalance
- poor development
- dysmenorrhea
- periodontal disease
- esophageal tear or rupture
- hair thinning
- bloating
- kidney damage
- potential fatality

TERMS	PRONOUNCIATIONS	DEFINITIONS
ehrlichiosis	(er-lik-e-o-sis)	a condition of tick bacterium infection characterized by malaise, fatigue, fever, listlessness, severe anemia, and hemoglobulinuria
emesis	(em-e-sis)	vomit or vomiting
encopresis	(en-ko-pre-sis)	fecal incontinence
eructation	(e-ruk-ta-shun)	belch or belching
feces	(fe-ses)	bowel waste, bowel movement, or BM
fissure	(fe-sur)	a crack in rectal or anal tissue
fistula	(fis-chu-la)	an abnormal pipe-like passageway
flatus or flatulence	(flay-tus)	gas
gastroenteritis	(gas-tro-en-ter-i-tis)	inflammation of the stomach and small intestine
gastroesophageal reflux or G.E.R.D.	(gas-tro-es-of-o-ge-al re-flux)	stomach and esophageal regurgitation causing burning and dyspepsia
Giardia	(gi-ar-de-a)	a parasitic illness of the small intestine
hernia	(her-ne-a)	a rupture or protrusion of an organ beyond its containment
intussusception	(in-tus-sus-sep-shun)	an intestinal telescoping that may cause an obstruction
irritable bowel syndrome or I.B.S.	(ir-rit-ab-el bow-el)	colonic spasm symptoms
metabolic syndrome or M.B.S. or syndrome x	(met-a-bol-ik)	syndrome x or a condition characterized by low LDL, heavy abdominal mid-section, high triglycerides, hyperglycemia, and hypertension
peristalsis	(per-is-tal-sis)	an involuntary rhythmic contraction
polyphagia	(pol-e-fa-ge-a)	excessive eating or swallowing
polyposis	(pol-e-po-sis)	condition of polyps or mushroom-like growths
postprandial	(post-pra-de-al)	related to after a meal
pyloric stenosis	(pi-lor-ik sten-o-sis)	a congenital narrowing of the stomach opening that may cause obstruction or projectile vomiting
reflux	(re-flux)	regurgitation of stomach contents (with dyspepsia and burning)
stoma	(sto-ma)	the site of an artificially established opening
syndrome x	(sin-drom x)	see metabolic syndrome
viscera	(vis-er-a)	internal organs

STUDY GUIDE: TESTS AND PROCEDURES

TERMS	PRONOUNCIATIONS	DEFINITIONS
anastomosis	(an-as-to-mo-sis)	artificially establishing an opening between two vessels or organs

TERMS	PRONOUNCIATIONS	DEFINITIONS
appendectomy	(a-pen-dek-to-me)	procedure or process of surgically removing the appendix
bariatric surgery	(bar-e-a-trik)	extreme surgical interventions focused upon weight reduction for the morbidly obese with health issues such as sleep apnea, asthma, type 2 diabetes, arthralgia/ exercise limitations, DVT, reflux, & unsuccessful weight loss with non-surgical interventions. Risks include anastomotic stricture, hernia, leaks, venous thrombosis, emboli, and a myriad of nutritional deficiencies
biliopancreatic diversion	(bil-e-o-pan-kre-at-ik di-ver-shun)	reduces the absorption of nutrients by bypassing most of the digestive tract (with or without a duodenal switch)
gastric bypass	(gas-trik by-pass)	upper stomach is stapled to allow only limited bypass
lap adjustable gastric banding	(lap ad-jus-tab-l gas-trik ban-ding)	a type of gastric bypass that offers an adjustable silicone band that is placed around the upper portion of the stomach
sleeve gastrectomy	(sev gas-trek-to-me)	process or procedure of surgical removal of 3/4 of the stomach
vertical banded gastroplasty	(ver-tik-al ban-ded gas-tro-plas-te)	process or procedure of reconstructing the stomach size with a band that essentially decreases the potential size of the stomach as well as its contents (15-30cc)
cholangiography	(ko-lanj-e-og-raf-e)	procedure or process of obtaining a radiopaque x-rays of cystic, hepatic, and common bile ducts
cholecystectomy	(kol-e-sis-tek-to-me)	procedure or process of surgically removing the gallbladder
colonoscopy	(kol-on-os-ko-pe)	procedure or process of examining the colon
colostomy	(ko-los-to-me)	procedure or process of artificially establishing a mouth-like opening in the colon
endoscopic retrograde cholangiopancreatography	(en-do-skop-ik ret-ro-grad kol-an-ge-o-pan-kre-at-o-graf-e)	examination of the biliary and pancreatic ducts via contrast media, scope, and film process
esophagogastroduodenalendoscopy	(e-sof-ago-gas-tro-du-od-en-al-end-os-ko-pe)	process of examination of the esophagus, stomach, and small intestine with biopsy, brushings, and/ or photographs
gastrectomy	(gas-trek-to-me)	procedure or process of surgically removing (a portion of) the stomach
gastrointestinal series or G.I. series	(gas-tro-in-tes-tin-al ser-ez)	barium and fluoroscopic GI examination

TERMS	PRONOUNCIATIONS	DEFINITIONS
gastrostomy	(gas-tros-to-me)	process or procedure of artificially establishing a mouthlike opening into the stomach
gavage	(ga-vaj)	feeding by nasogastric tube
halitosis	(hal-it-o-sis)	condition of foul breath
lavage	(la-vaj)	washing out or irrigation
occult blood	(o-kult)	fecal test for presence of blood
ova and parasites	(o-va)	fecal test for parasites and eggs
herniorrhaphy	(her-ne-or-a-fe)	procedure or process of surgical repair of a hernia
ileostomy	(il-e-os-to-me)	procedure or process of artificially establishing a mouth-like opening into the ileum
laparoscopy	(lap-ar-o-skop-e)	procedure or process of examining the abdomen and/ or an abdominal wall
laparotomy	(lap-ar-ot-o-me)	procedure or process of incising the abdomen and/or abdominal wall
lithotripsy	(lith-o-trip-se)	procedure or process of crushing or destroying stones

ABBREVIATIONS	DEFINITIONS
AC	before meals
BED	binge eating disorder
BM	bowel movement
BS	bowel sounds
ERCP	endoscopic retrograde cholangiopancreatography
GERD	gastroesophageal reflux disease
GI	gastrointestinal
HAV	hepatitis A virus
HBV	hepatitis B virus
HCV	hepatitis C virus
HDV	hepatitis D virus
HDL	high density lipoprotein
LDL	low density lipoprotein
IBS	irritable bowel syndrome
NBM	nothing by mouth
NG	nasogastric
NGTF	nasogastric tube feeding
NPO	nothing per os or nothing by mouth
N/V OR N&V	nausea and vomiting
O&P	ova and parasites
PC	after meals
PP or/ PRP	post prandial or after meals/preprandial or before meals
UGI	upper gastrointestinal

ABBREVIATIONS	DEFINITIONS
VH	viral hepatitis
WNL	within normal limits
jaundice	yellowish discoloration due to bile
icterus	yellowish skin, sclera, or other tissue discoloration

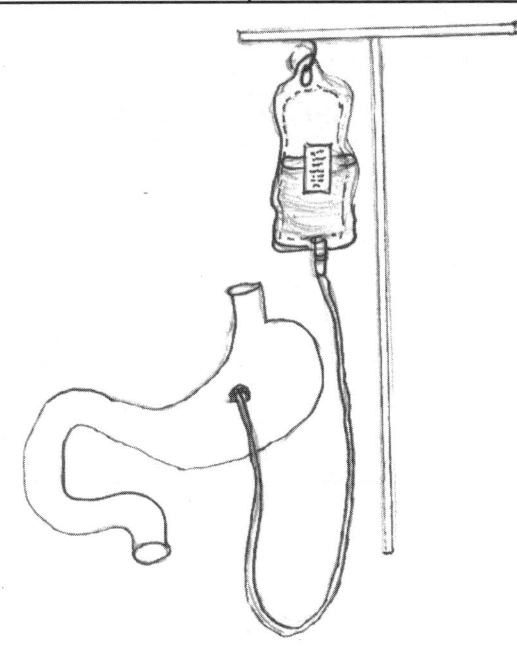

A gastrostomy for the purpose of feeding by tube

PRACTICE, PRACTICE, PRACTICE...........

Exercise 1:

As soon as you have received new medical terms, begin to review. Using blank 3"X5" index cards, create flashcards to review all of the new medical terms in this chapter by writing each of the correctly spelled terms five times on one side of the index card and the definition of each term on the other side of the index card. Keeping all of these cards in your right pocket, continually review all of the cards throughout the day. Whenever you have learned a card, place it in your left pocket. After you have learned all of these new terms, periodically refresh your memory with review.

Exercise 2:

Imagine That! Imagine that your family has a teenage member who has recently been diagnosed with an eating disorder. In writing; describe the adjustments you and your family would need to make socially, physically, emotionally, and financially. Next class, be prepared to informally share your findings with the class then hand in this written research paper using current professional resources.

Exercise 3:

Lightening Round Koosh Practice. With one or more study partners, throw a koosh ball to each other. The thrower poses a medical term from this chapter. The recipient is to correctly spell then define that term. The recipient always has the right to pass or call on another classmate for a life line assistance with the answer.

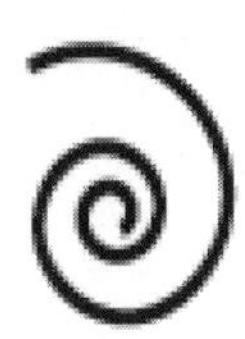

Chapter 15

Urinary System
The urinary or genitourinary system functions to filter and extract wastes from the blood.

STUDY GUIDE: ANATOMICAL

TERMS	PRONOUNCIATIONS	DEFINITIONS
kidney	(kid-nes)	an organ that excretes urine and purifies 1/4 of blood output
ureters	(yur-et-ers)	10-12" tubes that carry urine from the renal pelvis to the bladder
urethra	(yur-eth-ra)	the canal from the bladder that takes urine to the outside of the body
bladder	(blad-er)	an organ that holds urine
meatus	(me-at-us)	the extrenal opening to the outside of the body
anuria	(an-yur-e-a)	without urine
calculus	(kal-ku-lus)	stone (may cause severe pain and/or an obstruction). calculi=2 or more stones
diuresis	(di-yur-e-sis)	increase in urinary output
dysuria	(dis-yur-e-a)	related to difficult or painful urination
enuresis	(en-yur-e-sis)	bedwetting
frequency	(fre-kwen-se)	the urge to urinate often (more than once within 2 hours or 6-7 times within a day)
hematuria	(he-ma-tur-e-a)	related to blood in the urine
micturation or void	(mik-tur-a-shun)	urinate
nephrolithiasis or renal calculi	(nef-ro-lith-i-as-is)	condition of kidney stones
nocturia	(nok-tur-e-a)	related to night time urination
oliguria	(o-li-gur-e-a)	related to scanty urination
polyuria	(pol-e-yur-e-a)	related to excessive urination
pyuria	(pi-yur-e-a)	related to bacteria in urine
turbid	(tur-bid)	cloudy
urgency	(ur-jen-se)	extreme sensation of need to urinate
urine	(yur-in)	liquid evacuation from bladder
void or micturate	(voyd)	urinate

STUDY GUIDE: TESTS AND PROCEDURES

TERMS	PRONOUNCIATIONS	DEFINITIONS
catheterization	(kath-et-er-i-za-shun)	the process of using a flexible plastic tube (to empty the bladder, for example)
cystogram	(sis-to-gram)	x-ray of the bladder

TERMS	PRONOUNCIATIONS	DEFINITIONS
ystoscopy	(sis-tos-ko-pe)	procedure or process of examining the bladder
ialysis	(di-al-is-is)	process by which blood is artificially filtered
ithotripsy	(lith-o-trip-se)	procedure or process of crushing or destroying stones
enal transplant	(re-nal tranz-plant)	donor kidney surgically placed into recipient
rinalysis	(yur-in-al-is-is)	a clean caught urine specimen for general screening
rine culture	(yur-in kul-tur)	a sterile urine specimen to determine and identify any presence of bacteria

THE URINARY SYSTEM

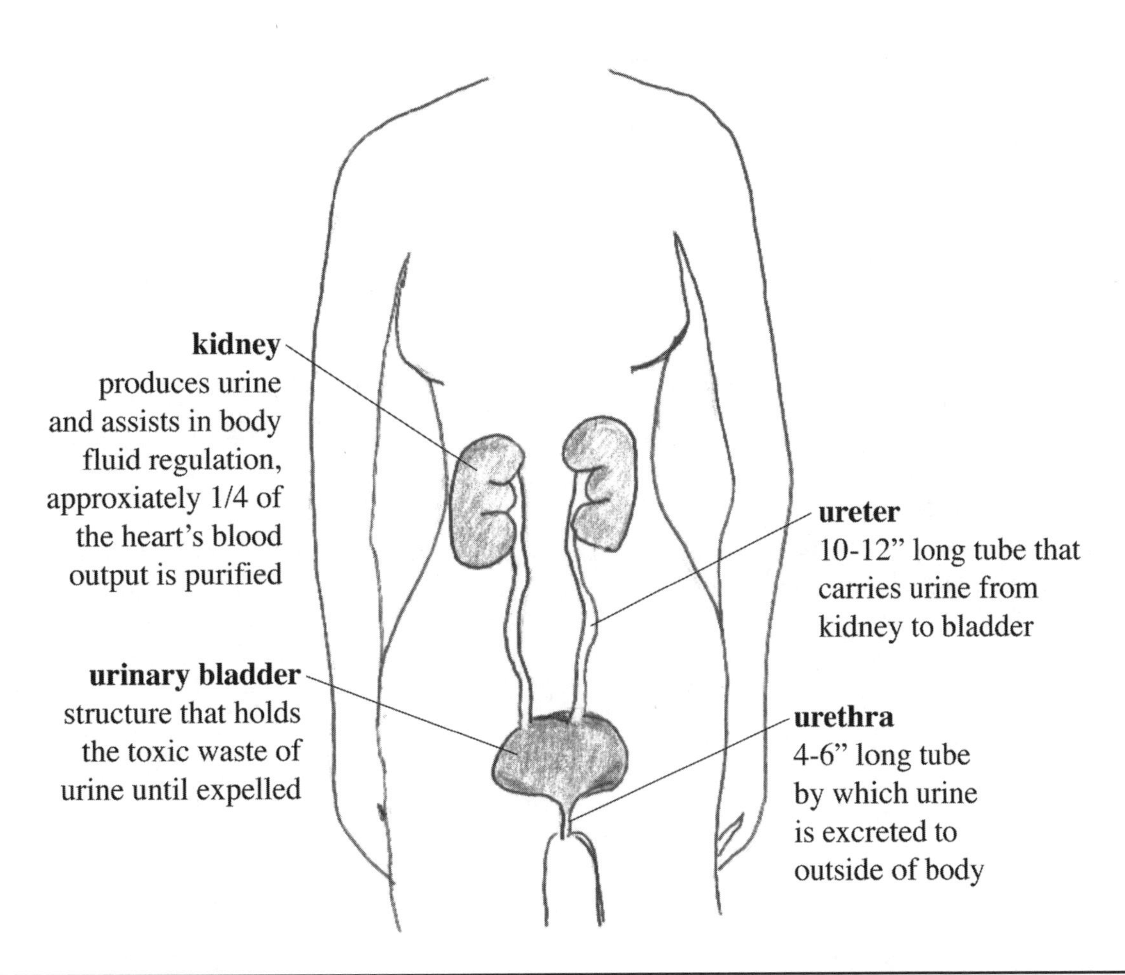

ABBREVIATIONS	DEFINITIONS
ARF	acute renal failure
BUN	blood urea nitrogen
CAPD	continuous ambulatory peritoneal dialysis
CATH	catheter or catheterization
CC	clean catch urine specimen or cubic centimeter

ABBREVIATIONS	DEFINITIONS
CRF	chronic renal failure
C&S	culture and sensitivity
ESRD	end stage renal disease
ESWL	extracorporeal shock wave lithotripsy
GU	genitourinary
HD	hemodialysis
I&O	24 hour intake and output record
IVP	intravenous pyelogram
K	potassium
Na	sodium
SG	specific gravity
NSU	non-specific urethritis
U/A or UA	urinalysis
U/C	urine culture
UTI	urinary tract infection

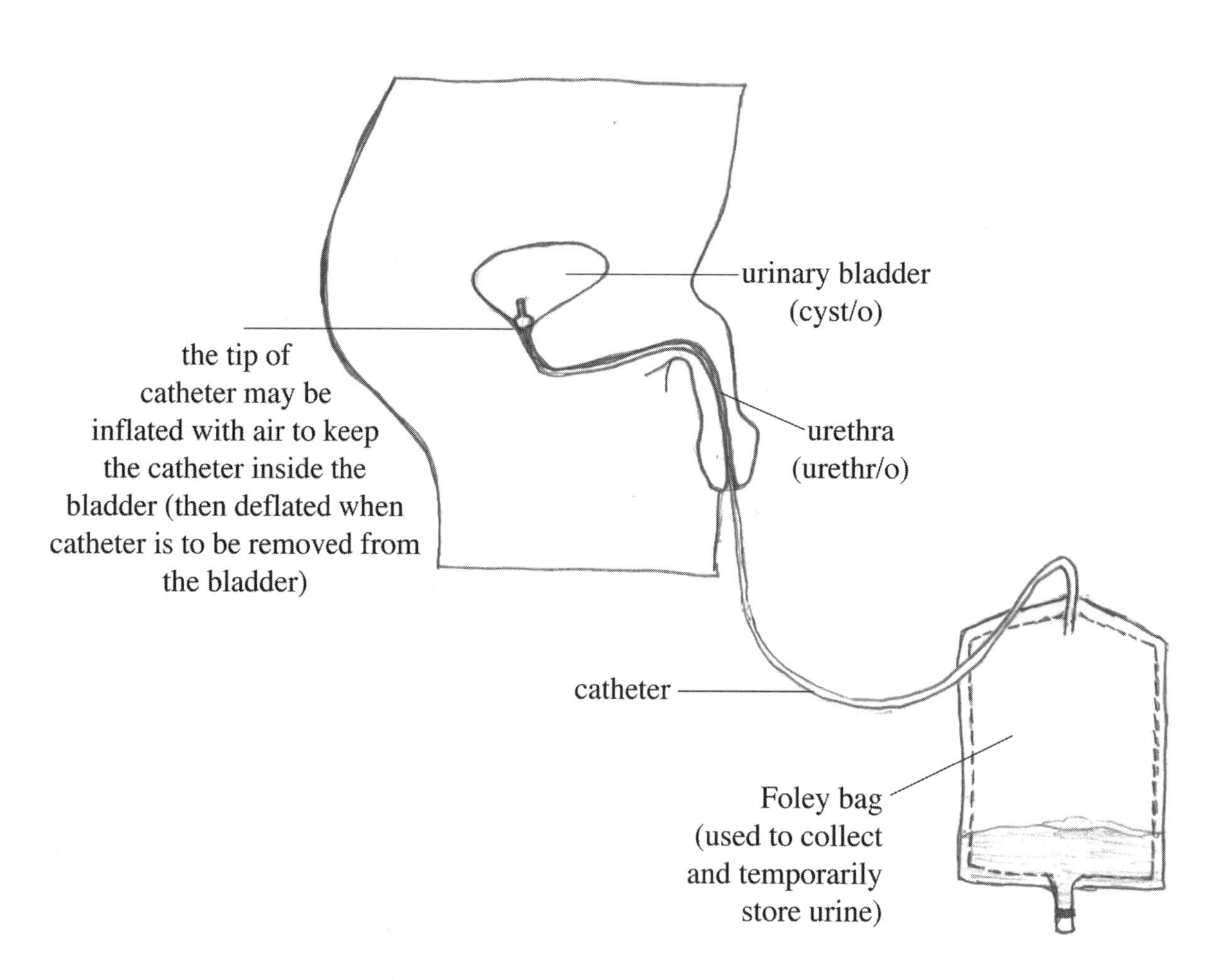

Urinary Catheterization: the process of using a flexible plastic tube to empty the bladder.

'RACTICE, PRACTICE, PRACTICE...........

:xercise 1:

.s soon as you have received new medical terms, begin to review. Using blank 3"X5" index cards, create flashcards to view all of the new medical terms in this chapter by writing each of the correctly spelled terms five times on one side of e index card and the definition of each term on the other side of the index card. Keeping all of these cards in your right ›cket, continually review all of the cards throughout the day. Whenever you have learned a card, place it in your left ›cket. After you have learned all of these new terms, periodically refresh your memory with review.

:xercise 2:

'eet the -Uria Family. List all of the medical term members possible from this family of the suffix -uria and then describe hat these terms stand for (definitions). For example: Meet anuria (no urine).

:xercise 3:

sing a compositional form, create an imaginary case history of a patient with cystitis incorporating a minimum of three ›breviations and ten medical terms from this chapter.

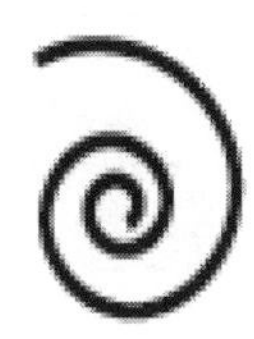

Chapter 16

Male Reproductive System
The male reproductive system produces sperm which may result in fertilization with an ovum.

STUDY GUIDE: ANATOMICAL

TERMS	PRONOUNCIATIONS	DEFINITIONS
testes	(tes-tez)	testicles, the male sex glands that produce sperm and secrete testosterone
epididymis	(ep-i-did-i-mis)	the ducts where sperm are stored
vas deferens	(vas def-er enz)	the testicular duct for excretion
seminal duct	(sem-in-al dukt)	the seminal vesicle duct for excretion
urethra	(yur-e-thra)	the tube that excretes urine and sperm to the exterior of the body
prostate	(pros-tat)	the gland surrounding the the urethra that secretes alkaline fluid
penis	(pe-nis)	muscular genitalia /sex organ containing erectile tissue
scrotum	(skro-tum)	the external sac containing the testis/ testes
prepuce	(pre-pus)	penal foreskin
genitalia	(jen-i-tal-e-a)	general male or female reproductive organs
aspermia	(a-sper-me-a)	without sperm
azoospermia	(a-zu-sperm-e-a)	related to semen without sperm
benign prostate hypertrophy or B.P.H.	(be-nin pros-tat)	prostate enlargement (not due to cancer)
carcinoma	(kar-sin-o-ma)	cancerous new growth, tumor, or neoplasm
condyloma acuminatum	(kon-dil-o-ma a-ku-min-a-tum)	HPV genital warts
cryptorchidism	(kript-ork-id-izm)	related to hidden or undescended testes (may lead to infertility)
epididymitis	(ep-i-did-i-mi-tis)	inflammation of the epididymis (causes inquinalgia and edema)
erectile dysfunction or E.D.	(e-rek-til dis-funk-shun)	inability to maintain an erection until ejaculation: impotence
impotent	(im-po-tent)	inability to maintain an erection until ejaculation: ED
phimosis	(fi-mo-sis)	condition of prepuce narrowing
pryotism	(pri-o-yizm)	related to prolonged tumescence (more than 4 hours)
seminoma	(sem-in-o-ma)	a testicular new growth, tumor, or neoplasm
spermatolysis	(sperm-at-o-li-sis)	sperm destruction

TERMS	PRONOUNCIATIONS	DEFINITIONS
umescence	(tu-mes-enz)	the process of becoming or being swollen (penal tumescence or erection)
varicocele	(var-i-ko-sel)	rupture, swelling, and/ or herniation veins (near testis)

THE MALE REPRODUCTIVE SYSTEM

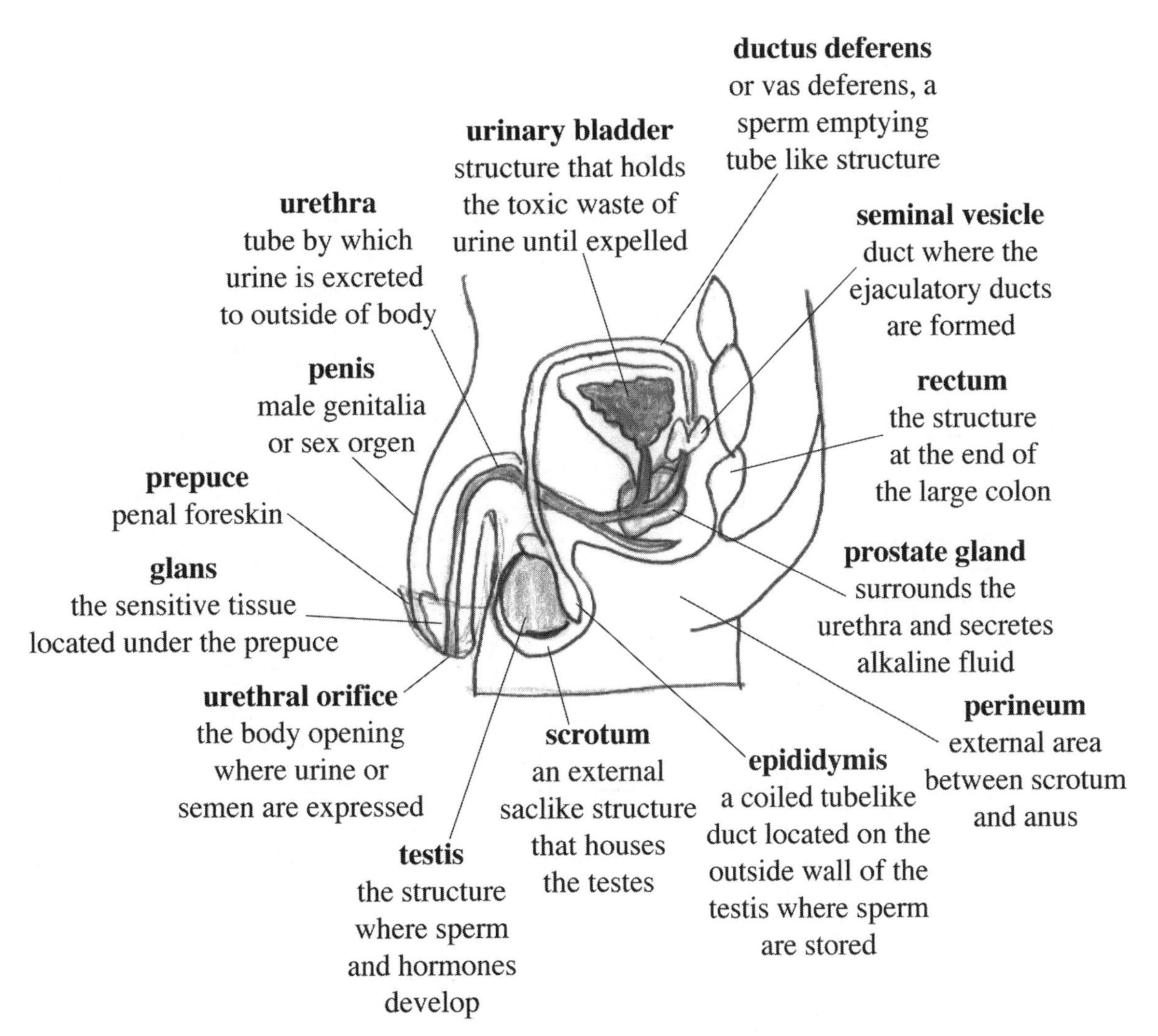

SEXUALLY TRANSMITTED DISEASE (STD)

TERMS	PRONOUNCIATIONS	DEFINITIONS
candida	(kan-di-da)	candidiasis or moniliasis condition
chlamydia	(kla-mid-e-a)	a very common asymptomatic but contagious bacterial infection
gonorrhea	(gon-or-e-a)	a communicable infection with urethral discharge
hepatitis B virus or H.B.V.	~	inflammation of the liver spread via bodily fluids
herpes simplex virus type 2 or HSV-2	~	a recurrent infection causing lesions

TERMS	PRONOUNCIATIONS	DEFINITIONS
human immunodeficiency virus or H.I.V.	~	a virus spread by bodily fluids that may cause infections, malignancies, and neurological issues
human papilloma virus or H.P.V.	~	a lesion causing virus spread by sexua contact and causes wart-like lesions
pediculosis pubis	(ped-ik-u-lo-sis pu-bus)	a condition of having pubic lice spreac by intimate exposure to a person infested
syphilis	(sif-il-is)	a contagious spirochete infection that may eventually involve any tissue or organ

STUDY GUIDE: PROCEDURAL

TERMS	PRONOUNCIATIONS	DEFINITIONS
brachytherapy	(brak-e-ther-ap-e)	implantation of internal radioactive isotopes to treat prostate cancer
circumcision	(sir-kum-si-shun)	related to cutting around the prepuce (foreskin excision)
digital rectal examination or D.R.E.	~	exam of the rectum via finger palpation
lumpectomy	(lump-ek-to-me)	procedure or process of surgical excision of a tumor, only (without any surrounding tissue or lymph nodes)
orchiectomy or orchidectomy	(or-ke-ek-t-o-me) or (or-kid-ek-to-me)	procedure or process of surgical excision of the testis or testes
orchiopexy	(or-ke-o-pex-e)	procedure or process of fixing testis into proper placement then suturing to secure this place
prostatectomy	(pros-ta-tek-to-me)	procedure or process of surgical excision or removal of the prostate
prostate-specific antigen test or P.S.A.	~	a blood screening test for pancreatic cancer
transurethral resection of the prostate or T.U.R.P.	(tranz-yur-e-thral)	prostate gland removal through the urethra
urethrogram	(yur-eth-ro-gram)	prostate and urethral x-ray picture
vasectomy	(vas-ek-to-me)	procedure or process of surgical excision or removal of part of the vas deferens (male sterilization)
vasovasostomy	(vas-o-vas-os-to-me)	a vasectomy reversal involving reopening and reattaching of the vas deferens

ABBREVIATIONS	DEFINITIONS
AIDS	acquired immune deficient syndrome (end stage HIV)
AIH	artificial insemination, homologous
ARC	AIDS-related complex

ABBREVIATIONS	DEFINITIONS
BPH	benign prostate hypertrophy
DRE	digital rectal examination
ED	erectile dysfunction
ELISA	HIV screening test
HBV	hepatitis B virus
HIV	human immunodeficiency virus
HPV	human papilloma virus
HRT	hormone replacement therapy
HSV-2	herpes simplex virus type 2
NSU	non-specific urethritis
KS	Kaposi's sarcoma
PSA	prostate-specific antigen
STD	sexually transmitted disease
TSE	testicular self exam
TUR or TURP	transurethral resection of the prostate
VD	venereal disease

PRACTICE, PRACTICE, PRACTICE...........

Exercise 1:

As soon as you have received new medical terms, begin to review. Using blank 3"X5" index cards, create flashcards to review all of the new medical terms in this chapter by writing each of the correctly spelled terms five times on one side of the index card and the definition of each term on the other side of the index card. Keeping all of these cards in your right pocket, continually review all of the cards throughout the day. Whenever you have learned a card, place it in your left pocket. After you have learned all of these new terms, periodically refresh your memory with review.

Exercise 2:

Sell It. Create a commercial for an imaginary new drug to treat the condition of your choice (include a minimum of ten medical terms from this chapter).

Exercise 3:

Fill in the Blank.

When he was 3 y/o, Mr. Smith had undescended testes or ____________________ which was surgically corrected with an ____________________. P.H. also revealed Hx of ________________ (a S.T.D.) and a ____________________ (the male sterilization procedure). Currently, Mr. Smith presents with an abnormal outcome on a test of antigen that is prostate specific (also known as a ______________ test). The ___________________ (specialist in male/ reproductive issues) has recommended a ______________________ (a picture or recording of the prostate and urethra) as well as ____________________ (process of implanting radioactive isotopes). Dx:______________________.

ANSWER KEY: cryptorchidism, orchiopexy, H.P.V. (or any other S.T.D.), vasectomy, PSA, urologist, urethrogram, brachytherapy, urethritis

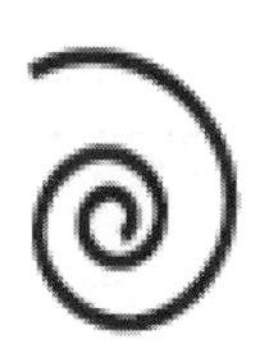

Chapter 17

Female Reproductive System
The female reproductive system produces ovum which may result in fertilization with a sperm.

STUDY GUIDE: ANATOMICAL

TERMS	PRONOUNCIATIONS	DEFINITIONS
areola	(ar-e-o-la)	area of darker pigmentation surrounding the nipple
Bartholin's glands	(bar-tho-lin)	2 glands on either side of the vagina that secrete lubrication upon stimulation
breast	(brest)	sensory and/or hormonally dictated lactation apparatus
cervical os	(ser-vik-al os)	the cervical opening at the lower end of the uterus
cervix	(ser-viks)	the lower neck-like areas of the uterus
clitoris	(klit-o-ris)	a small vulvalar female organ containing erectile tissue
endometrium	(en-do-me-tre-um)	the inner part of the uterine wall
fallopian tubes	(fa-lo-e-an)	the ducts wherein fertilization usually occurs and where ovum is transported from the ovary to the uterus
fundus	(fun-dus)	the upper portion of the uterus
gamete	(gam-et)	an ovum or a spermatozoon (a mature reproductive cell)
hymen	(hi-men)	a thin mucous membrane that encircle the external vaginal opening
introitus	(in-troy-tus)	entrance to the vaginal cavity
labia majora	(la-be-a ma-jor-a)	the larger lip-like skin fold in the opening of the female genitalia
labia minora	(la-be-a min-or-a)	the smaller lip-like skin fold that protects the clitoris
meatus	(me-a-tus)	opening
orifice	(or-if-is)	opening to a cavity (vaginal orifice)
ovaries	(o-var-ez)	female sex glands where the ova are produced
ovum (or ova)	(o-vum) or (o-va)	egg (or 2 or more eggs)
perineum	(per-i-ne-um)	the region located from the introitus to the anus
uterus	(u-ter-us)	a pear shaped organ in the middle of the pelvis wherein a placenta is formed during pregnancy
vagina	(va-ji-na)	2 1/2-4" long muscular tube from the cervix to the exterior body
vulva	(vul-va)	external female genitalia

TERMS	PRONOUNCIATIONS	DEFINITIONS
zygote	(zi-got)	a fertilized egg

STUDY GUIDE:

TERMS	PRONOUNCIATIONS	DEFINITIONS
abruptio placenta	(a-brup-te-a pla-sen-ta)	early (before the 20th week of pregnancy) separation of a normally positioned placenta
breech	(brech)	delivery presentation of feet or buttocks first
contraction	(kon-trak-shun)	involuntary rhythmic labor process by which the fetus and placenta are expelled
crowning	(krow-ning)	the baby's head is positioned where it is externally visable in the vaginal birth canal
dyspareunia	(dis-par-u-ne-a)	related to difficult or painful sexual intercourse
dysplasia	(dis-pla-se-a)	related to difficult or painful cellular growth
dystocia	(dis-to-she-a)	related to difficult or painful labor
eclampsia	(e-klamp-se-a)	a pregnancy complication of toxemia or pregnancy induced hypertension with seizures (potentially fatal)
ectopic	(ek-top-ik)	related to pregnancy outside of the uterus (often in the fallopian tube)
effacement	(e-fas-ment)	the active labor process in which the cervix dilates partially and shortens prior to the transition to full dilation
embryo	(em-bre-o)	the term for fertilization from third to eighth week of life
fetus	(fe-tus)	the term for fertilization from the ninth week until delivery
forceps (a tool) or vacuum suction (a process)	(for-seps)	assistive delivery tool for (or process of) removal of the fetus from the vaginal canal
gestation	(jes-ta-shun)	the pregnancy period from conception to birth
gravida	(gra-vid-a)	pregnancy
lactation	(lak-ta-shun)	mammary gland secretion of breast milk following childbirth
meconium	(mek-o-ne-um)	the newborn's first stool (usually resembles black tar)
menarche	(men-ar-ke)	menstrual onset
menstruation	(men-stru-a-shun)	menstrual flow secondary to lack of conception
menopause	(men-o-pawz)	menstrual cessation
menorrhagia	(men-or-aj-e-a)	related to excessive bursting forth of menstrual bleeding
multigravida or GRAV-2 (or more)	(mul-te-grav-id-a)	more than one pregnancy

TERMS	PRONOUNCIATIONS	DEFINITIONS
nulligravida or GRAV-O	(nul-e-grav-id-a)	no pregnancy
primigravida or GRAV-1	(prim-i-par-a)	one or first pregnancy
perimenopause	(per-i-men-o-pawz)	the period around the cessation of menstruation
multipara	(mul-ti-par-a)	more than one live birth
neonate	(ne-o-nat)	newborn: birth to four weeks of age
nullipara	(nul-i-par-a)	no live birth
primipara	(prim-i-par-a)	one or first live birth
parturition	(par-tu-ri-shun)	childbirth
perineum	(per-i-ne-um)	the area from the anus to the vagina
placenta	(pla-sen-ta)	the structure that nourishes the fetus, the afterbirth
placenta previa	(pla-sen-ta pre-ve-a)	the placenta blocks the birth canal by relocating to the lower uterus
polydactylism	(pol-e-dak-til-izm)	related to more than five digits on the hand or foot
pre-eclampsia	(pre-e-klamp-se-a)	a potentially fatal complication of pregnancy characterized by weight gain, edema, hypertension albuminuria, and/or headache (may lead to toxemia)
presentation	(pre-en-ta-shun)	the position of the infant in the uterus before delivery
toxemia	(tox-em-e-a)	eclampsia or pregnancy induced hypertension with seizures
trimester	(tri-mes-ter)	the 3: three month periods of the gestational time
umbilical cord	(um-bil-ik-al)	the means of placental attachment to the fetus
vernix caseosa	(ver-nix ka-se-o-sa)	the exterior cheese-like substance protecting the newborn prior to delivery
viable	(vi-a-bul)	capable of survival on its own

STUDY GUIDE: TESTS AND PROCEDURES

TERMS	PRONOUNCIATIONS	DEFINITIONS
abortion, A.B., ab, or T.A.B.	(ab-or-shun)	related to the process of miscarriage or expulsion of the material related to conception prior to development of a viable fetus (termination of a pregnancy)
amniocentesis	(am-ne-o-sen-te-sis)	abdominal needle aspiration of amniotic fluid for diagnostic evaluation of genetic issues
Apgar	(ap-gar)	a 10 point numerical score given post-delivery assessing a newborn's physical condition at 1 minute and 5 minutes for color, pulse, responsiveness, movement, and respirations

TERMS	PRONOUNCIATIONS	DEFINITIONS
aspiration biopsy	(as-pir-a-shun)	withdrawal of tissue and/ or fluid for the process of examination of living cells (cytology)
cervical conization	(ser-vik-al ko-ni-za-shun)	related to the process of removing triangular cone shaped cervical tissue for cellular examination
cesarean, c-section, or CS	(ses-ar-e-an)	a surgically assited delivery via the abdomen and uterus
chorionic villus sampling or C.V.S.	(kor-e-on-ik vil-us)	vaginal catheterization for withdrawal of chorionic cells from placental tissue (to rule out genetic defects)
colporrhaphy	(kolp-or-af-e)	procedure or process of surgically repairing the vagina
colposcopy	(kolp-os-ko-pe)	procedure or process of vaginal examination with an instrument
cryosurgery	(kri-o-sur-jer-e)	procedure or process of surgically removing tissue by freezing the abnormal tissue
dilation and curettage or d&c	~	cervical widening or dilation and endometrial scraping or curettage to remove or obtain tissue as well as to control bleeding
embolization	(em-bo-li-za-shun)	process by which beads of plastic or gelatin sponge are injected via a catheter to the uterine artery to block small arteries and prevent blood supply to fibroid tumors (to shrink the fibroids)
episiotomy	(ep-es-e-ot-o-me)	procedure or process of making a perineal incision (to assist delivery and prevent an anal laceration)
gamete intrafallopian transfer or G.I.F.T.	(gam-et)	assisted fertilation technique recommended for women with intact fallopian tubes (eggs are retreived by laparoscope then natural fertilization occurs in the fallopian tubes)
hysterectomy	(his-er-ek-to-me)	procedure or process of surgical excision of the uterus
immobilization	(im-o-bil-i-za-shun)	process or procedure of blocking blood supply to shrink a tumor
induction	(in-duk-shun)	cervical stimulation to encourage vaginal delivery
in vitro fertilization or I.V.F.	(in-ve-tro)	fertilization that is assisted outside of the body

STUDY GUIDE: PROCEDURAL

TERMS	PRONOUNCIATIONS	DEFINTIONS
mammogram	(mam-o-gram)	picture or recording of the breast
oophorectomy	(of-or-ek-to-me)	procedure or process of surgical excision of an ovary

TERMS	PRONOUNCIATIONS	DEFINITIONS
large-loop excision of the transformation zone or L.L.E.T.Z.	~	a device used to treat precancerous cervical lesions via simultaneous excision, biopsy, and treatment in between the endocervix and the ectocervix (eg; the transformative zone, where abnormal cells tend to form)
loop electrosurgical excision procedure or L.E.E.P.	~	an electrosurgical device used to simultaneously excise, biopsy, and treat abnormal cervical lesions (dysplasia or HPV)
ableration	(ab-ler-a-shun)	a procedure of laser destruction of uterine lining
embolization	(em-bo-li-za-shun)	process of stopping or blocking blood flow (fibroids)
pelvimetry	(pel-vim-e-tre)	procedure or process of measuring the diameter of the pelvis
salpingoophorectomy	(sal-ping-of-or-ek-to-me)	procedure or process of surgical excision of the fallopian tubes and the ovary/ovaries
salpingostomy	(sal-ping-os-to-me)	procedure or process of artificially establishing an opening in the fallopian tube
stereotactic surgery	(ster-e-o-tak-tik)	the process of mimally invasive surgery including biopsy, ablation, implantation, stimulation, lesion injection, and radio surgery

ANTERIOR PERSPECTIVE OF INTERNAL FEMALE REPRODUCTIVE SYSTEM

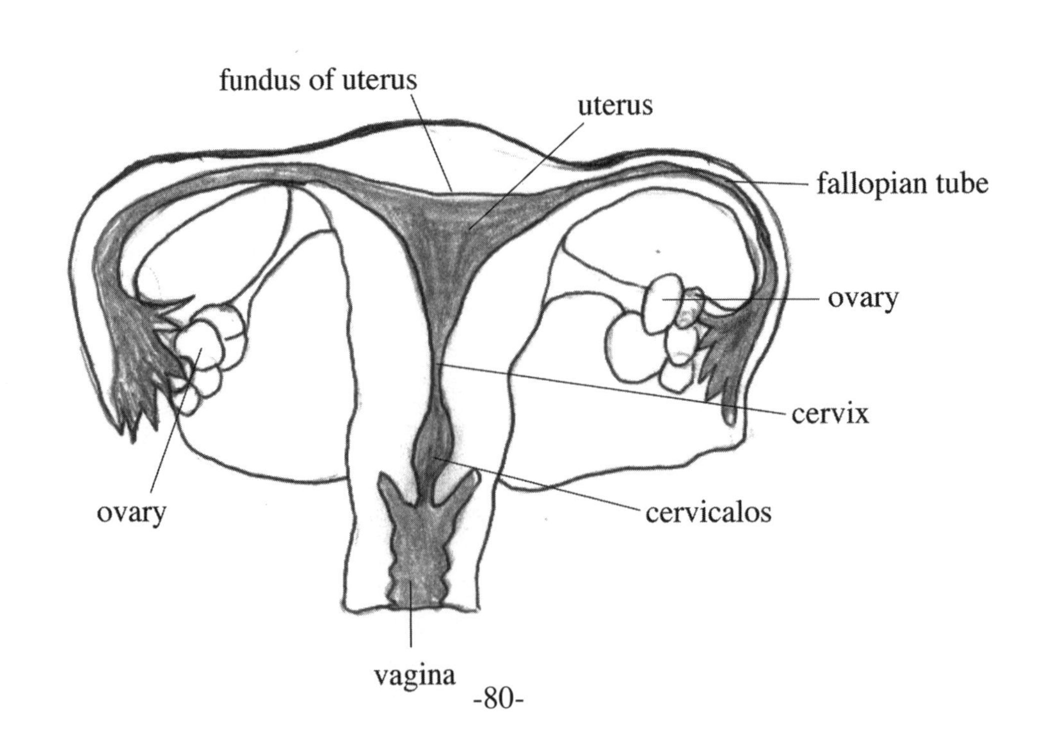

ABBREVIATIONS	DEFINITIONS
AB, ab, or TAB	abortion or therapeutic abortion
AFP	alpha fetaprotein blood test during pregnancy
BSE	breast self examination
BSO	bilateral salpingoophorectomy
BWS	battered woman syndrome
C-SECTION or CS	cesarean
CVS	chorionic villus sampling
Cx	cervix
D&C	dilation and curettage of uterine lining
EDD	estimated date of delivery
EFM	electronic fetal monitor
ELECTRZ	treatment for cervical dysplasia
ERT	estrogen replacement therapy
FHR	fetal heart rate
FHT	fetal heart tone
FTND	full term or normal delivery
GARD	Gardasil, a vaccine to help protect against HPV (and throat or cervical cancer)
GDM	gestational diabetes mellitus
GIFT	gamete intrafallopian transfer
GYN	gynecology
GRAV-1	one or first pregnancy, primigravida
HRT	hormone replacement therapy
IUD	intrauterine device
IVF	in vitro fertilization
L&D	labor and delivery
LEEP	loop electrosurgical excision procedure
LLETZ	large-loop excision of the transformation zone
LMP	last menstrual period
ND	normal delivery
OB/GYN	obstetrics/gynecology
OCP	oral contraceptive pills
PAP	PAP smear
PID	pelvic inflammatory disease
PMS	premenstrual syndrome
SAB	spontaneous abortion
SVD	spontaneous vaginal delivery
TAB	therapeutic abortion
TSS	toxic shock syndrome
UAE	uterine artery immobilization (blocks blood supply to tumor)
VBAC	vaginal birth after cesarean

ABBREVIATIONS	DEFINITIONS
VH	vaginal hysterectomy
ZIFT	zygote intrafallopian transfer

SAGITTAL PERSPECTIVE OF FEMALE PELVIC REGION

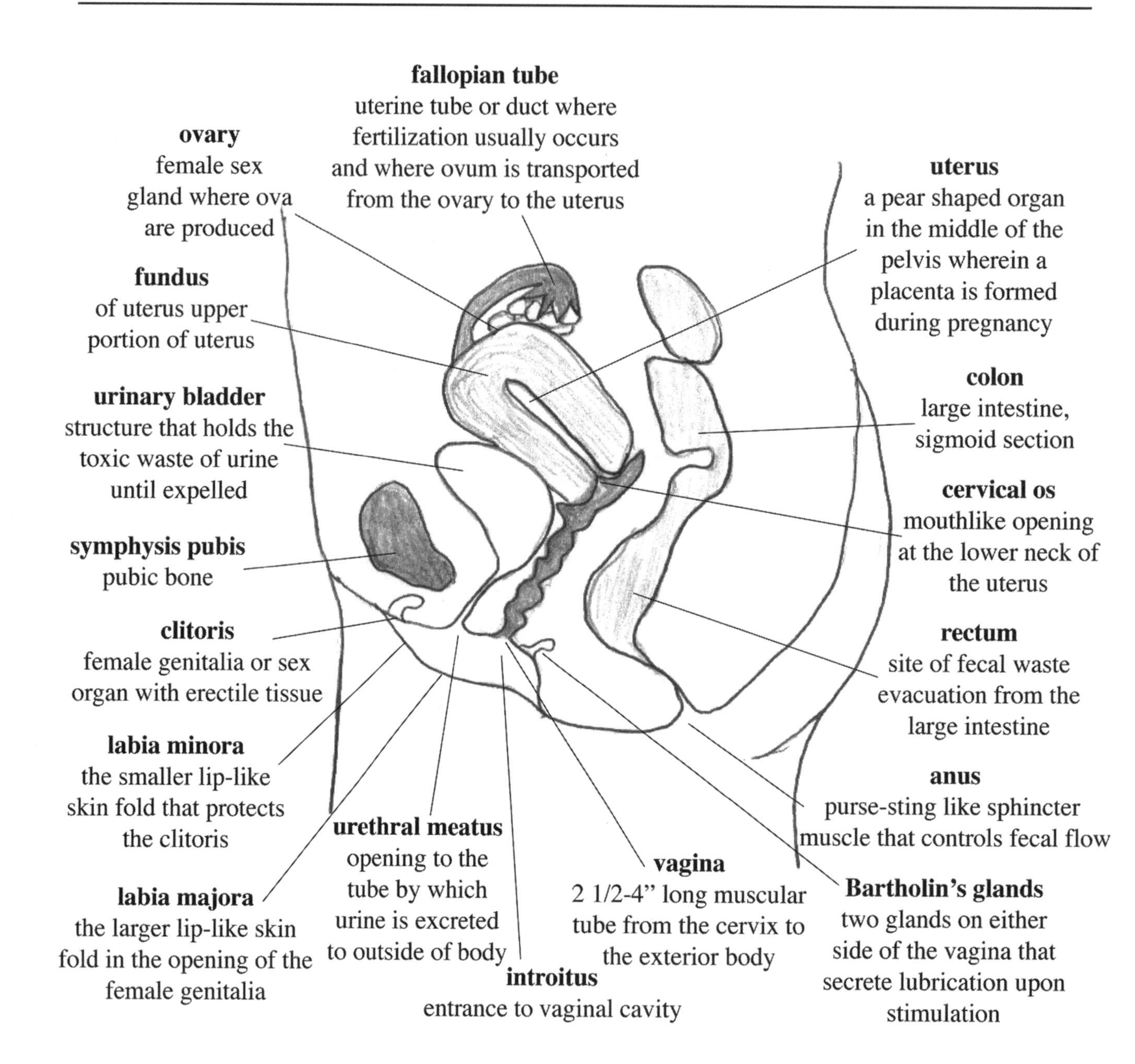

PRACTICE, PRACTICE, PRACTICE...........

Exercise 1:

As soon as you have received new medical terms, begin to review. Using blank 3"X5" index cards, create flashcards to review all of the new medical terms in this chapter by writing each of the correctly spelled terms five times on one side of the index card and the definition of each term on the other side of the index card. Keeping all of these cards in your right pocket, continually review all of the cards throughout the day. Whenever you have learned a card, place it in your left pocket. After you have learned all of these new terms, periodically refresh your memory with review.

xercise 2:

ıld Card. Utilize your individual strengths to present a memorable review of this chapter (or at least 20 terms) to your ıssmates at the next scheduled class. For example; if you are computer savvy; prepare a Power Point C.D..If you are ›atrical, create a skit. If you are musically gifted, set a song to medical term lyrics. If you are a writer, make a limmerick a poem involving medical terms. If you are artistic, sketch or paint your visual conception of these terms. If you are a ker, prepare a food to share with the class that illustrates these terms. This exercise may be approached individually or concert with others in order to divide and conquer this task.

xercise 3:

›ws Flash Report to Class: Report any three current, professional advances germane to any topic from this chapter as ›ll as one little known fact.

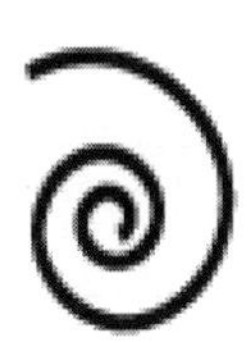

Chapter 18

Sensory Receptors: Eyes, Ears, and Mouth
The eyes function as sensory receptors for vision, the ears for hearing as well as equilibrium, and the mouth for taste.

STUDY GUIDE: ANATOMICAL EYE

TERMS	PRONOUNCIATIONS	DEFINITIONS
sclera	(skler-a)	the outer covering of the eyeball
conjunctiva	(kon-junk-ti-va)	the mucous membrane that covers an protects the eyeballs as well as eyelid
iris	(i-ris)	the colored band around the pupil and cornea
pupil	(pu-pil)	the hole in the center of the iris that regulates the pupil size to accommodate for light
lens	(lenz)	a transparent structure that refracts light rays
aqueous humor	(a-kwe-us)	the clear fluid in front of the anterior lens chamber
vitreous humor	(vit-re-us)	the transparent gelatinous-like materi in the eyeball
optic nerve	(op-tik)	related to the nerve for sending retina images to the brain
macula	(mak-u-la)	retinal center
retina	(ret-in-a)	receptor for images produced by the lens (contains nerve cells like the rods and cones)
rods	(rods)	light sensitive nerve cells enabling dim, black, and white imagery
cones	(kons)	light sensitive nerve cells enabling bright and colored imagery
accomodation	(a-kom-o-da-shun)	ability to adjust eyes for distance
amblyopia	(am-ble-o-pe-a)	related to dull, dim, or weak vision
atosmia	(ar-os-me-a)	no sense of smell
astigmatism	(a-stig-ma-tizm)	without even eye focus causing visual disturbance
blephoroptosis	(blef-or-op-to-sis)	upper eyelid drooping
dacryorrhea	(dak-re-or-e-a)	excessive tear secretion
diabetic retinopathy	(DR)	process of retinal damage due to diabetes (visual blind spots and loss)
enucleation	(e-nuk-le-a-shun)	surgical eyeball removal
esotropia	(e-so-tro-pe-a)	eye(s) and vision turn(s) inward toward nose
exotropia	(x-o-tro-pe-a)	eye(s) and vision turn(s) outward toward temples
hyperopia	(hi-per-o-pe-a)	farsightedness

TERMS	PRONOUNCIATIONS	DEFINITIONS
nyopia	(mi-op-e-a)	nearsightedness
resbyopia	(pres-be-op-e-a)	visual change associated with aging
mmetropia	(em-e-tro-pe-a)	normal vision
laucoma	(glaw-ko-ma)	increased intraocular pressure that may lead to blindness (generally asymptomatic in early development but then incurs increasing loss of peripheral vision)
rachoma	(tra-ko-ma)	chronic bacterial disease common in dry climates that may lead to blindness (conjunctivitis and corneal inflammation)
ataract	(kat-ar-akt)	increasingly opaque and cloudy lens that leads to blindness
acrimation	(lak-rim-a-shun)	related to tear production
nacular degeneration	(MD)	loss of central vision with aging
ystagmus	(nis-tag-mus)	rapid, left to right or right to left eye movement (characteristic of an inner ear or nervous system issue)
ptic	(op-tik)	related to vision or eyes
phthalmologist	(of-thal-mol-o-jist)	specialist in the science or study of the eye
ptician	(op-tish-an)	specialist in eye products
optometrist	(op-tom-e-trist)	specialist in measuring and fitting eye wear
otolaryngologist	(ot-o-lar-in-gol-o-gist)	ear and voice box specialist (ENT)
photophobia	(fo-to-fo-be-a)	related to sensitivity or pain with light exposure
strabismus	(stra-bis-mus)	eye muscle misalignment
stye or hordeolum	(sti or hor-de-ole-um)	an acute eyelid infection of the sebacious gland

EYE ABBREVIATIONS	DEFINITIONS
ACC	accommodation
ARMD	age-related macular degeneration
As	astigmatism
cgl	correction with glasses
E	eye
EM	emmetropia or normal vision
EOM	extraocular movement
ERG	electroretinography
ET	esotropia
EX	exotropia
H, hy	hyperopia, farsightedness
LASIK	laser-assisted in situ keratomileusis
L&A	light and accommodation

EYE ABBREVIATIONS	DEFINITIONS
M, my	myopia
NREM	non rapid eye movement (sleep)
OD or RE	right eye
OS or LE	left eye
OU	both eyes
PERLA or PERRLA	pupils equal and reactive (responsive) to light accomodation
REM	rapid eye movement
VA	visual acuity
+	plus, positive, or convex
-	minus, negative, or concave

VISION

The passage of light rays from an object through the cornea, aqueous humor, lens and vitreous humor to the retina.

emmetropia
(normal vision)

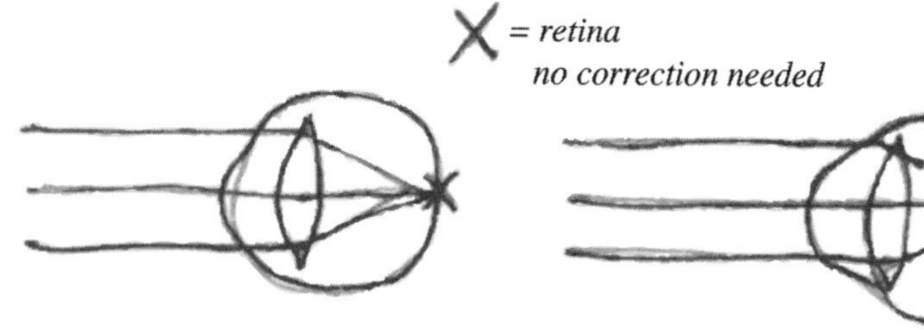

At a distance of six meters or more, light rays are brought to a focus on the retina by the lens.

myopia
(nearsightedness)

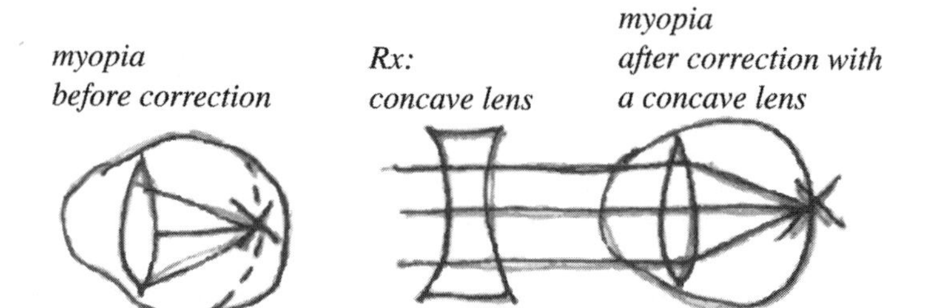

At the distance of six meters or more, light rays are brought to a focus in front of the retina.

hyperopia
(farsightedness)

hyperopia
before correction

Rx:
convex lens

hyperopia
after correction with
a convex lens

At a distance of six meters or more, light rays are brought to a focus in back of the retina.

esotropia
(eye(s) and vision turn inward toward the nose)

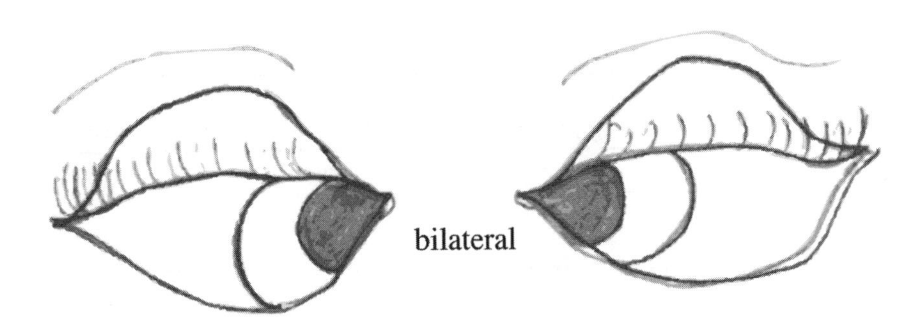

exotropia
(eye(s) and vision turn outward toward the temples)

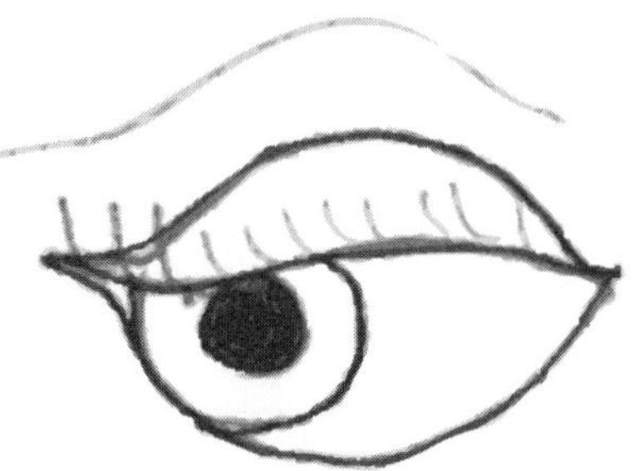

bilateral

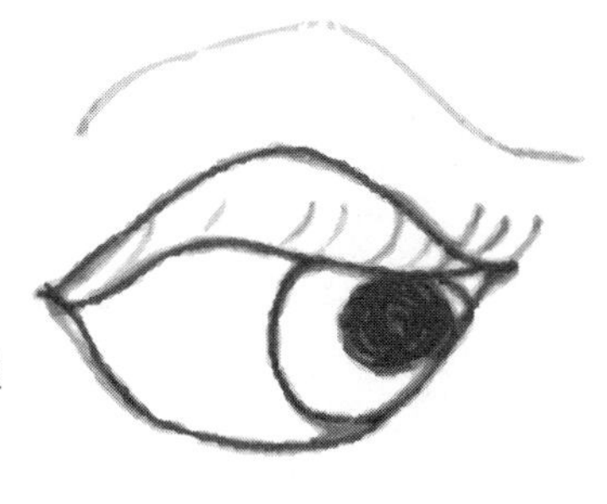

TUDY GUIDE: ANATOMICAL EAR

TERMS		PRONOUNCIATIONS	DEFINITIONS
xternal ear:	auricle or pinna	(ar-ik-el or pin-a)	funnel-shaped ear flap that collects sound
	auditory meatus	(awd-itor-e me-a-tus)	ear canal
niddle ear:	tympanic membrane	(tim-pan-ik mem-bran)	TM (eardrum)
	ossicles	(os-ik-els)	ear bones (smallest body bones)
nner ear:	vestibule	(ves-ti-bul)	vibration collection area
	semicircular canals	(semi-sirk-u-lar kan-als)	hearing and equilibrium
	cochlea	(ko-kle-a)	sensory receptor
	eustachian tube	(ew-sta-shun tub)	tube between pharynx and middle ear
coustic		(a-kus-tik)	related to hearing
uditory		(aw-di-tor-e)	related to hearing
erumen		(ser-u-men)	ear wax (located in the auditory meatus)
xternal otitis		(x-ter-nal o-ti-tis)	an external fungal or bacterial inflammation of the auditory meatus characterized by itching or tenderness
xudate		(x-u-dat)	bacterial or cellular drainage secondary to infection
mastoiditis		(mas-toyd-i-tis)	inflammation of the mastoid process
Meniere's disease		(men-e-ars)	a chronic and progressive syndrome (characterized by vertigo, otalgia, and tinnitus)
myringotomy		(mi-ring-ot-o-me)	procedure or process of making an incision into tympanic membrane
otic		(o-tik)	related to ears
otitis media		(o-ti-tis)	middle ear infection
otolaryngologist (or ENT)		(o-to-lar-in-gol-o-jist)	specialist of ears to voice box

TERMS	PRONOUNCIATIONS	DEFINITIONS
otoplasty	(ot-o-plas-te)	procedure or process of ear reconstruction
otosclerosis	(ot-o-skler-o-sis)	condition of hardening of the ear
otoscope	(ot-o-skop)	lighted instrument used to examine th ear
otoscopy	(ot-o-skop-e)	procedure or process of examining the ear
presbycusis	(pre-be-o-pe-a)	nerve damage and/or hearing loss due to aging
pressure-equalizing tubes	(PE tubes)	tubes inserted following a myringotomy to promote air flow into the eustachian tube, prevent otitis media, and assist drainage
tinnitus	(tin-i-tus)	internal auditory noises (ringing, whooshing, buzzing)
tympanotomy	(tim-pan-ot-o-me)	procedure or process of incising the eardrum (TM)
tympanoplasty	(tim-pan-o-plas-te)	procedure or process of middle ear reconstruction (to correct a rupture or perforation)
vertigo	(ver-ti-go)	dizziness

EAR ABBREVIATIONS	DEFINITIONS
AD	right ear
AS	left ear
AU	both ears
db	decibel
ENT	ear, nose, throat
EENT	ear, eye, nose, throat
AOM	acute otitis media
OM	otitis media
BOM	bilateral otitis media
SOM	serous otitis media
ORL	otorhinolaryngology
PET	pressure equalizing tubes
TM	tympanic membrane

STUDY GUIDE: MOUTH ANATOMICAL

TERMS	PRONOUNCIATIONS	DEFINITIONS
bicuspids	(bi-kus-pids)	premolars
cuspids	(kus-pids)	anterior canine teeth
gingiva	(ji-jiv-a)	gum or soft tissue encircling the tooth
incisors	(in-siz-or)	front cutting teeth
molars	(mo-lars)	posterior teeth

MOUTH TERMS	PRONOUNCIATIONS	DEFINITIONS
nodontia	(an-o-dot-e-a)	related to without teeth
ruxism	(brux-izm)	nightime teeth-grinding
alculus	(kal-ku-lus)	plaque or tooth tartar (stone like)
aries	(kar-ez)	cavities secondary to tooh decay
entalgia	(den-tal-ge-a)	tooth pain
entist	(den-tist)	tooth specialists
ysgeusia	(dis-ge-se-a)	difficult sense of taste
ndodontist	(en-do-don-tist)	specialist in pulp and related tissues
xodontia	(x-o-don-te-a)	related to tooth extraction
orensic dentist	(for-en-zik)	specialist related to identifying dental remains
eriodontist	(jer-e-o-don-tist)	specialist in dentistry of the elderly
ustation	(gus-ta-shun)	sense of taste
nalocclusion	(mal-o-klu-shun)	misalignment
dontalgia	(o-dont-al-ge-a)	related to tooth pain
rthodontist	(or-tho-don-tist)	specialist in tooth alignment
alate	(pal-at)	roof of the mouth
edodontist	(ped-o-don-tist)	specialist in children's dentistry
eriodontist	(per-i-o-don-tist)	specialist in the tissues around the teeth
rosthodontist	(pros-tho-don-tist)	specialist in the formation of artificial tooth appliances or devices
yorrhea	(pi-or-e-a)	bacterial flow of discharge
emporomandibular joint disorder	(TMJ)	a joint misalignment condition
TMJ	~	temporomandibular joint disorder

RACTICE, PRACTICE, PRACTICE..........

xercise 1:

s soon as you have received new medical terms, begin to review. Using blank 3"X5" index cards, create flashcards to eview all of the new medical terms in this chapter by writing each of the correctly spelled terms five times on one side of e index card and the definition of each term on the other side of the index card. Keeping all of these cards in your right ocket, continually review all of the cards throughout the day. Whenever you have learned a card, place it in your left ocket. After you have learned all of these new terms, periodically refresh your memory with review.

xercise 2:

lphabet Soup. Students with last names starting with A-G, create a replica of two eyeballs. Students with last names tarting with H-P, make representations of two ears. Students with last names starting with Q-Z, show us an open mouth odel. Guidelines: all presentations should be three dimensional, clearly illustrate a minimum of five medical conditions s well as five anatomical terms, and be thoughtfully executed in a size/scale that is conducive to classroom illustration.

xercise 3:

ickle the Terminology. Research any ten medical terms from this chapter for the purpose of uncovering funny, quirky, or ttle known factoids about them. Be prepared to share your findings with the class then hand them in next meeting. The urpose of this exercise is to assist recall of medical terminology presented this chapter.

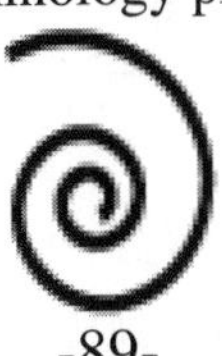

Chapter 19

The Endocrine System and The Stress Response
The endocrine system regulates metabolism via ductless gland secretions. In concert with the nervous system, the endocrine system promotes homeostasis.

STUDY GUIDE: ANATOMICAL

TERMS	PRONOUNCIATIONS	DEFINITIONS
adrenal glands	(a-dren-al glans)	secretes stressbusting hormones, assists metabolism, and regulates fluids/ electrolytes
diabetes insipidus	(di-a-be-tes in-sip-i-dus)	inadequate ADH pituitary secretion (sx: polyuria and polydipsia)
diabetes mellitus	(di-a-be-tes mel-i-tus)	disorder of carbohhydrate/ glucose metabolism (hyperglycemia and glycosuria) - a disease in which the body does not produce or ineffectively uses the produced insulin (a hormone secreted by the pancreas and needed to convert sugar/ glucose and carbohydrates into energy) - the increase in obesity in the U.S is highly correlated with the increased incidence of diabetes. - when insulin is not properly used; glucose builds up in the blood and can contribute to vessel hardening, retinopathy, slowed healing process, hypercholestemia, hypertension, stroke, and/or heart disease - follow-up recommendations include smoking cessation, weight loss, cholesterol control, B/P monitoring, a controlled diet (low glucose, carbohydrates, transfat, salt, saturated fat, and cholesterol), fasting blood glucose monitoring, regular podiatrist examinations, ophthalmological follow-up, regular aerobic exercise, appropriate stress management and adequate daily rest
pre-diabetes (mellitus) or P.D.M.	~	a fasting blood glucose of 100-125mg/ dL
diabetes mellitus, type 1 or T.I.D.M.	~	the pancreas produces little or no insulin (daily injection or infusion required for survival)

TERMS	PRONOUNCIATIONS	DEFINITIONS
diabetes mellitus, type 2 or T2DM	~	the pancreas makes too little insulin or cannot efficiently utilize whatever insulin it makes (also known as insulin resistance)
gestational diabetes or GDM	~	pregnancy induced diabetes mellitus
hyperglycemia	(hi-per-gli-se-me-a)	too little insulin and too much blood glucose that may lead to ketoacidosis/ diabetic coma Sx: polyphagia, glycosuria polydipsia, paresis polyuria, weight loss nocturia, fatigue blurred vision, retinopathy neuropathy
hypoglycemia	(hi-po-gli-se-me-a)	too much insulin and too low blood glucose that may lead to insulin shock Sx:vertigo,confusion, and nervousness
pancreas	(pan-kre-as)	secretes insulin as well as regulates glucose and starch
parathyroid glands	(par-a-thi-royd)	maintains calcium and phosphorous levels
pineal gland	(pin-e-al)	makes seratonin as well as regulates circadian rhythm, sexual development, and mood
pituitary gland	(pi-tu-it-ar-e)	produces growth and other hormones (that regulate the other glands)
sex glands	(sex glans)	testes and ovaries stimulates sexual development
thymus	(thi-mus)	supports immunity and lymphoid tissue
thyroid gland	(thi-royd)	maintains metabolism
acidosis	(a-sid-o-sis)	condition of acidity or carbon dioxide accumulation within body fluids
ketosis	(ke-to-sis)	condition of ketone accumulation due to insufficient fatty acid metabolism
ketoacidosis, K.A., or D.K.A.	(ke-to-a-sid-o-sis)	condition of abnormal presence of ketone bodies in the blood and urine signaling poor carbohydrate metabolism, starvation, and/ or poor diabetes management
metabolic syndrome, MBS, or syndrome x	~	a syndrome of insulin resistence/ T2DM, obesity, hypertension
polydipsia	(pol-e-dip-se-a)	related to excessive thirst
polyphagia	(pol-e-fa-ge-a)	related to excessive eating/swallowing
nocturia	(nok-tur-e-a)	related to getting up at night to urinate
glycosuria	(gli-ko-sur-e-a)	related to glucose (sugar) in urine

TERMS	PRONOUNCIATIONS	DEFINITIONS
polyuria	(pol-e-yur-e-a)	related to excessive urination
neuropathy	(ner-o-path-e)	process of any disease of the nerves
retinopathy	(ret-in-o-path-e)	process of any disease of the retina
diaphoresis	(di-a-for-e-sis)	profuse perspiration
acromegaly	(a-kro-meg-al-e)	a disorder or process of enlargement of the head, feet, hands, and face due to excessive somatotropin secretion
Addison's disease	(ad-i-sons)	adrenal hyposecretion characterized by paresis and/ or weight loss
Cushing's disease	(kush-ings)	adrenal hypersecretion characterized by edema, paresis, skin discoloration, porous bones, and/ or excessive hair growth
Grave's disease	(gravs di-ez)	thyroid hypersecretion, hyperthyroidism, goiter, and lack of iodine
Hashimoto's disease	(hash-i-mo-tos)	chronic thyroidism, an autoimmune disorder
hirsutism	(hir-su-tizm)	condition of excessive hair
hypercholestemia	(hi-per-ko-les-te-me-a)	high cholesterol in blood
hyperthyroidism	(hi-perthi-royd-izm)	excessive thyroid secretion and increased metabolic rate
hypothyroidism	(hi-po-thi-royd-izm)	under active metabolism and thyroid secretion
metabolism	(met-ab-o-lizm)	the process by which ingested nutrients are converted to heat and other general energy
metabolic syndrome, MBS, or syndrome x	(met-a bol-ik)	hyperglycemia caused by insulin resistance and often associated with hypercholestemia,, obesity, low HDL, hypertension, and/ or heart disease

STRESS TERMS	DEFINITIONS
homeostasis	the body's tendency to maintain the same balanced internal environment at a state of relaxation and health
stress response	the physiological sympathetic nervous system response to a stressor
stressor	any real or perceived as if real pressure that results in a sympathetic response
parasympathetic response	the nervous system that activates the relaxation response
eustress	relaxation after the stressor has passed (helps body to manage stressors in a healthy way)
sympathetic response	the physical 'fight or flight' response to a stressor (the stress response)
distress	a prolonged sympathetic response after the stressor has passed (that may contribute to a myriad of illnesses)
target organ	the physical area or organ affected by distress

STRESS TERMS	DEFINITIONS
tress management techniques	strategies designed to prevent stressors or to assist in healthy coping with stressors
rganization	documentation and planning ahead
neditation	prolonged quiet period of inwardly focused thought for the purpose of relaxation and mental clarity
RONTO plan	prevent procrastination and panic by immediate action and scheduled reinforcements by putting aside plenty of time to regroup and refresh (with artistic projects, pampering, exercise, meditation, etc.)
umor	never underestimate the power of laughter as a physiological benefit
elf talk	tell yourself positive messages and "take the reins" for making your life wonderful starting with what you say to you
R & R	rest, relax, nourish, and care for yourself everyday
isualization	positive and luxurious imagery used to focus on for the purpose of relaxation
rogressive muscle relaxation (PMR) and/or exercise	an exercise incorporating toe to head maximum muscular tension to induce maximum body relaxation. All reasonable exercise is generally a beneficial and health promoting activity.

THE STRESS RESPONSE

stressor = any real or imagined pressure, force or strain that results in a sympathetic response

sympathetic = nervous system response that activates "fight or flight" for stressor survival

distress = bad stress as unable to relax after the stressor is over. It is a prolonged sympathetic response that contributes toward poor health

parasympathetic = nervous system response that activates relaxation

eustress = good stress that helps body cope w/ stressors then relaxes after stressor is over promotes good health

homeostasis

homeostasis = relaxation or your body's tendency to maintain its individual internal health and calmness

ABBREVIATIONS	DEFINITIONS
A1c	glycated hemoglobin (long term glucose control blood test)
ACTH	adrenocorticotropic hormone
ADH	antidiuretic hormone
CGM	continuous glucose monitoring
DI	diabetes insipidus

ABBREVIATIONS	DEFINITIONS
DKA	diabetic ketoacidosis
DM	diabetes mellitus
FBS	fasting blood sugar
FSH	follicle stimulating hormone
GH	growth hormone
GTT	glucose tolerance test
IDDM	insulin dependent diabetes mellitus
JOD	juvenile onset diabetes
LH	lutenizing hormone
Na	sodium
NIDDM	non-insulin dependent diabetes mellitus
OXT	oxytocin
PBI	protein bound iodine test (measures blood thyroxine)
PRL	prolactin
RAIU	radioactive iodine uptake test
RIA	radioimmunoassay test (measures blood hormone levels)
T1DM	type 1, diabetes mellitus
T2DM	type 2, diabetes mellitus
T3	triodothyronine
T4	thyroxine
T7	free thyroxine index
TFT	thyroid function test
TSH	thyroid-stimulating hormone

PRACTICE, PRACTICE, PRACTICE..........

Exercise 1:

As soon as you have received new medical terms, begin to review. Using blank 3"X5" index cards, create flashcards to review all of the new medical terms in this chapter by writing each of the correctly spelled terms five times on one side of the index card and the definition of each term on the other side of the index card. Keeping all of these cards in your right pocket, continually review all of the cards throughout the day. Whenever you have learned a card, place it in your left pocket. After you have learned all of these new terms, periodically refresh your memory with review.

Exercise 2:

Walk a Mile in Other's Mocassins. As a class group or individually, imagine that you are the parent of twin ten year old girls and an eight year old boy. The endocrinologist has just diagnosed your son with type 1 diabetes mellitus. What will you need to address socially, physically, emotionally, and financially in order to help your family adjust successfully to the news? What specific adjustments will need to be addressed in school, over holidays, at home, when on field trips or overnights, etc. Brainstorm and write out your care plan.

Exercise 3:

What's New? Research the roles played by obesity and distress in the development of Syndrome X. Write a one page explanation of your findings and why they are important. Be prepared to review and creatively sell your prevention message to your target audience (your classmates) next class.

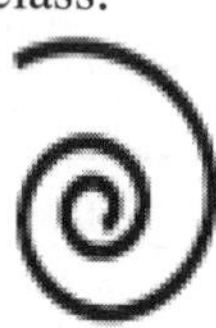

Chapter 20

'ervous System

'he nervous system is comprised of the central nervous system, the peripheral ervous system, and the autonomic nervous system. The central nervous ystem (the brain and the spinal cord) and the peripheral nervous system the cranial and the spinal nerves) regulate most voluntary or consciously ontrolled functions. The autonomic nervous system (the ganglia and the erves) regulates most involuntary or unconsciously controlled functions. 'ogether with the endocrine system, the nervous system assists in maintaining 'omeostasis.

ANATOMICAL TERMS	PRONOUNCIATIONS	DEFINITIONS
›rain	(brayn)	contains the cerebrum (voluntary motor motion, eyesight, consciousness, sensations, and emotions), the cerebellum (coordination, equilibrium, and posture), and the brain stem (respirations, heart beat, blood vessel dilation and constriction)
›pinal cord	(spi-nal kord)	acts as conduction between brain and bodily impulses as well as the seat of the reflexes
neninges	(me-nin-jes)	brain and spinal cord membranes
:erebrospinal fluid or C.S.F.	(ser-eb-ro-spi-nal flew-id)	fluid that encircles and cushions the brain and spinal cord
:ranial nerves	(kra-ne-al)	the twelve pairs of nerves (coming from the cranium)
›lfactory	(ol-fak-tor-e)	sense of smell process
›ptic	(op-tik)	related to vision or sense of sight
›culomotor	(ok-u-lo-motor)	eyelid muscle and pupil movement
rochlear	(trok-le-ar)	eyeball muscle
:rigeminal	(tri-jem-in-al)	jaw, facial, nose, mouth, and forehead muscles (related to)
ıbducens	(ab-du-sens)	lateral eyeball muscles
facial	(fa-shal)	expressive face, ear, and scalp muscle
ıcoustic or auditory	(a-kus-tik)	sense of hearing process
glossopharyngeal	(glos-o-far-in-ge-al)	related to taste and swallowing, tongue and throat
vagus	(va-gus)	voice and abdominal muscles
spinal	(spi-nal)	related to spine
ıypoglossal or sublinqual	(hi-po-glos-al)	related to under the tongue
sympathetic nervous system	(sim-pa-thet-ik)	produces the "fight or flight" stress response (increases heart rate, respirations, and metabolic rate; dilates bronchi and pupils; and decreases gastrointestinal functioning)

ANATOMICAL TERMS	PRONOUNCIATIONS	DEFINITIONS
parasympathetic nervous system	~	produces relaxation and eustress (decreases respirations and heart rate, increases GI function, and constricts bronchi as well as pupils)

TERMS	PRONOUNCIATIONS	DEFINITIONS
agnosia	(ag-nos-e-a)	although generally functioning, without knowing or ability to identify objects or sounds
akinesia	(a-kin-es-e-a)	related to being without voluntary motion
amyotrophic lateral sclerosis or A.L.S.	(am-e-o-trof-ik lat-er-al skler-o-sis)	a condition of hardening characterized by a progressive deterioration of functioning and early ataxia (also called Lou Gehrig's disease)
Alzheimer's disease	(al-zi-mers)	a chronic disorder characterized by progressive mental deterioration, disorientation, apathy, speech issues, memory loss, judgement impairment, issues of physical orientation, and other neurodegenerative disturbances
aneurysm	(an-yur-ism)	a weakened, dilated, and ballooned part of a vessel (that may rupture)
aphagia	(a-fa-ge-a)	related to without eating or swallowing
aphasia	(a-fa-ze-a)	related to without speech
apraxia	(a-prax-e-a)	related to without ability to conduct motor activity
asthenia	(as-the-ne-a)	related to loss of strength
ataxia	(a-tax-e-a)	related to without muscular coordination
atonia	(a-to-ne-a)	related to without muscular tone
autism	(aw-tizm)	impairment in social interaction
Bell's palsy	(bals pal-se)	process of temporary one-sided facial paralysis
bradykinesia	(bra-de-kin-es-e-a)	related to slow voluntary movement
cerebral palsy	(ser-a-bral pal-se)	process of postural and movement abnormalities due to early brain development issues
craniomalacia	(kran-i-o-mal-a-se-a)	related to softening of the skull bones
dysarthria	(dis-arth-re-a)	related to difficulty with speech articulation
dysfluency	(dis-flu-en-se)	process of difficult repetition of syllable/phrase
dyslexia	(dis-lex-e-a)	related to difficult or different comprehension or application of language
epilepsy	(ep-il-ep-se)	process of a chronic brain disorder characterized by seizures and loss of consciousness

TERMS	PRONOUNCIATIONS	DEFINITIONS
rand mal	(grand mal)	a type of epileptic seizure involving sudden loss of consciousness and tonic muscular contractions
uillain-Barr	(ge-ya-bar-a)	a syndrome involving sudden paresis, reflex response loss, and poor neural impulses that often occur 1-3 weeks after an acute viral infection
erpes zoster or shingles	(her-pez-zos-ter)	an acute viral condition
yme disease	(lim dis-ez)	a multiple-system disorder caused by a spirochete from a deer tick, sx: circular rash at bite site, fatigue, chills, fever, headache, myalgia, arthralgia or enlarged lymph nodes
etite mal	(pe-tet mal)	a type of epileptic seizure involving a milder and briefer epileptic seizure that resembles daydreaming
emiparesis	(hem-i-par-e-sis)	half or one-sided remarkable/weakness
emiplegia	(hem-i-plej-e-a)	half or one-sided paralysis
ethargy	(leth-ar-ge)	process of sluggishness
lasticity	(plas-ti-sit-e)	the theoretical process that the brain can relearn or adapt through repetition (following neurological issues)

AREAS OF BRAIN FUNCTIONING

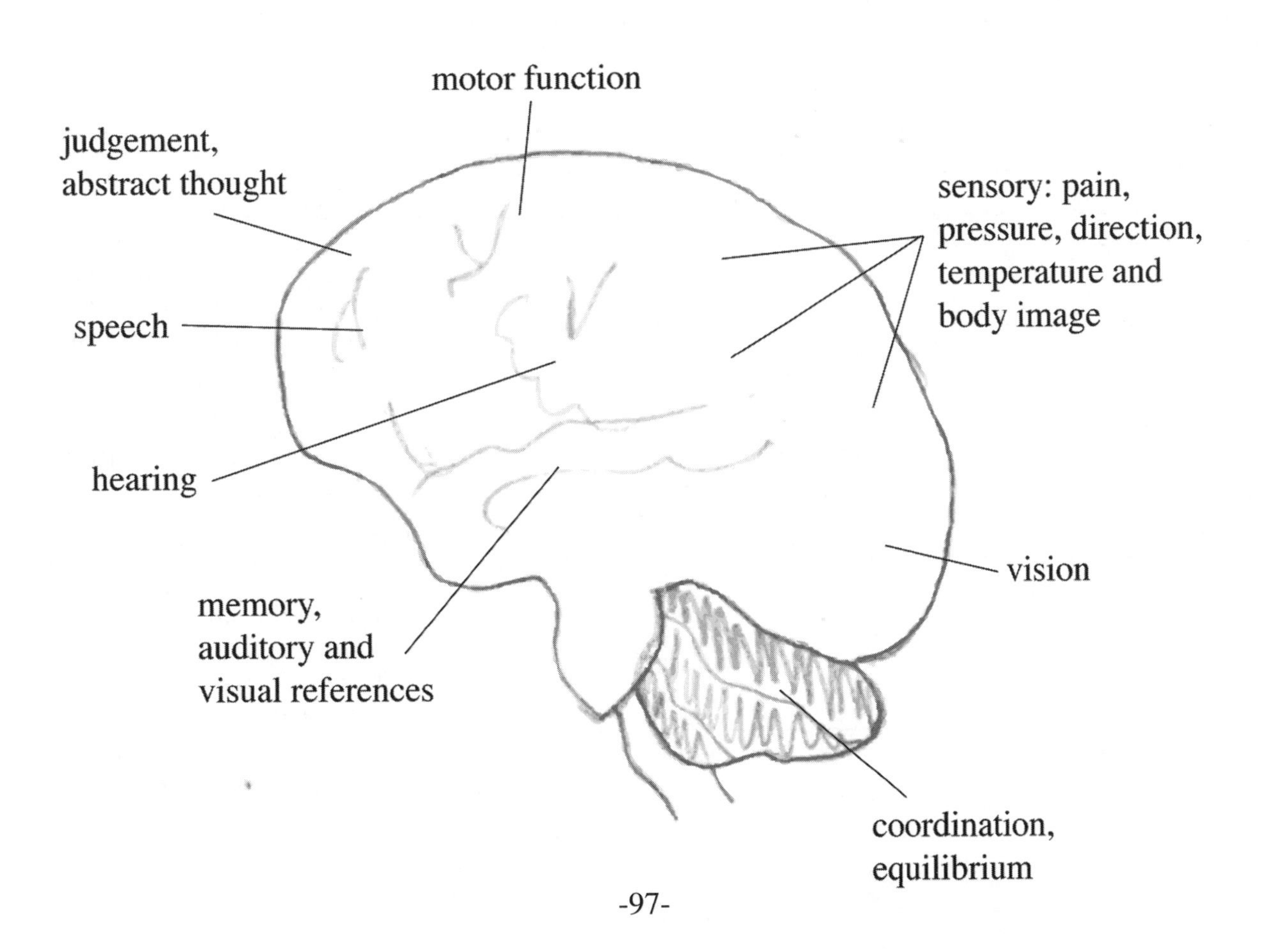

****

Know the 911:

TERMS	PRONOUNCIATIONS	DEFINITIONS
meningitis	(men-in-ji-tis)	inflammation of the meninges characterized by sudden stiff neck, headache, nausea, or fever (viral or bacterial, contagious & may be fatal)
Moya Moya disease	(moy-a moy-a)	a progressive occlusion of tiny internal vessels in the carotid artery (unknown cause often associated with meningitis, Franconi's anemia, brain atherosclerosis, vasculitis, and some genetic issues). Sx include: TIA (possibly with seizures) or CVA
multiple sclerosis or M.S.	(mul-ti-pul skler-o-sis)	condition of a chronic inflammatory disease involving many areas of grey matter hardening which results in numbness, tremor, poor coordination, paresis, speech issues, visual disturbances, & other neurological issues
myasthenia gravis or M.G.	(mi-as-the-ne-a grav-is)	related to a chronic disease characterized by fatigue and paresis
narcolepsy	(nar-ko-lep-se)	chronic process involving involuntar episodes of sleeping (with REM)
nystagmus	(nis-tag-mus)	involuntary rapid eye movement of the eyeball with impaired coordinatio that may affect walking and standing
obtunded	~	a patient with dulled or diminished mental capacity due to a trauma or condition
paraplegia	(par-a-ple-ge-a)	related to paralysis of the lower body
paresis	(par-e-sis)	remarkable weakness
Parkinson's disease	(par-kin-sons)	a chronic nervous system disorder characterized by shuffling gait, paresis, frustration, muscular rigidly, poor equilibrium, tremors, and nausea
pica	(pi-ka)	an eating disorder characterized by craving for non-food material
postictal	(post-ik-tal)	confusion following a seizure
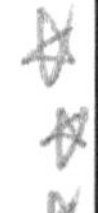 quadriparesis	(kwa-dri-par-e-sis)	remarkable weakness of all four limbs
quadriplegia	(kwa-dri-ple-ge-a)	paralysis of all four limbs
Reye's syndrome	(rayz)	an acute disorder involving hypoglycemia, brain edema, intracranial pressure, and other vital organ issues (viral or caused by ingestion of Aspirin by a child)
shingles or herpes zoster	(shin-gels)	an acute viral condition involving a painful vesicle eruption along the nerve pathway of the body trunk

TERMS	PRONOUNCIATIONS	DEFINITIONS
syncope	(sin-ko-pe)	fainting or temporary loss of consciousness
Tourette's syndrome	(tur-ets)	a genetic disorder characterized by facial tics and/or utterances that may be obscene
Wernicke's encephalopathy	(wer-nik-ez en-sef-al-op-ath-e)	any disease process of the brain and meninges caused by thiamine deficiency or chronic alcoholism, sx: delirium, tremors, visual changes or mental confusion with disorientation
stroke	(strok)	brain tissue death due to insufficient blood O2
EMERGENCY immediate medical assistance required (brain tissue dies within minutes of blood supply interruption)		
transient ischemic attack or T.I.A.	(tran-se-ent is-kem-ik at-ak)	a miniature stroke in which the blood supply within a vessel lumen leading to the brain narrows or becomes blocked with plaque (usually occurs in 5-20 minutes) Sx may include: - sudden hemiparesis of face, arm, & leg - denial - sudden hemiplegia - imbalance, vertigo - sudden numbness (usually on one side) or loss of grasp - dysphagia - visual disturbance or impairment - aphagia - difficulty with judgement, decision making, or understanding - dystaxia - mental confusion suddenly - ataxia - general anxiety - dysphasia - gait change or sudden walking issue - aphasia
cerebrovascular accident (CVA)	(ser-e-bro-vas-ku-lar ax-i-dent)	a hemorrhagic stroke.(sx: sudden, severe headache) with unknown cause)

If one or more of these signs, IMMEDIATELY CALL 9-1-1.
Questions? Call the American Stroke Association 1-888-4-STROKE
or contact their website: http://www.americanstroke.org/

****

LYME DISEASE - CARRYING TICK SIZES

1) Adult Male Tick 2-2.7mm

2) Nymph Tick 1.3-1.7mm

3) Larvae 0.7-0.8mm

ABBREVIATIONS	DEFINITIONS
AD	Alzheimer's disease
A&O	'alert and oriented' following a mental status check
ALS	amyotropic lateral sclerosis or Lou Gehrig's disease
ANS	autonomic nervous system
CAT	computerized axial tomography
CNS	central nervous system
CP	cerebral palsy
CSF	cerebrospinal fluid
CVA	cerebrovascular accident
EEG	electroencephalogram
EMG	electromyogram
LP	lumbar puncture or spinal tap
MRI	magnetic resonance imaging
MS	multiple sclerosis
NREM	non-rapid eye movement
PET	positron emission tomography
PNS	peripheral nervous system
REM	rapid eye movement
TENS	transcutaneous electrical nerve stimulation
TIA	transient ischemic attack

Know the differences between ataxia, apraxia, atrophy, aplasia, aphasia, aphagia, and aphonia.

PRACTICE, PRACTICE, PRACTICE...........

Exercise 1:

As soon as you have received new medical terms, begin to review. Using blank 3"X5" index cards, create flashcards to review all of the new medical terms in this chapter by writing each of the correctly spelled terms five times on one side o the index card and the definition of each term on the other side of the index card. Keeping all of these cards in your right pocket, continually review all of the cards throughout the day. Whenever you have learned a card, place it in your left pocket. After you have learned all of these new terms, periodically refresh your memory with review.

Exercise 2:

Watch T.V., find a video, D.V.D., or television show that illustrates any medical term related to the nervous system and write a one page synopsis of what you witnessed.

Exercise 3:

Poster Project. Using outside resources, create a diagram showing your understanding of any medical condition related t the nervous system for the purpose of teaching others about it.

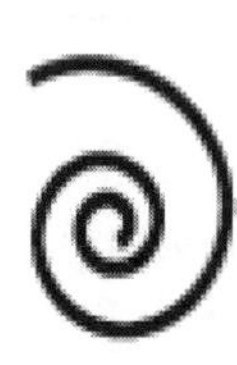

Chapter 21

Psychiatric Terms

This chapter encompasses terms related to medical compliance and psychological issues that may interfere with daily healthy functioning.

STUDY GUIDE:

TERMS	PRONOUNCIATIONS	DEFINITIONS
affect	(a-fekt)	general emotional reaction
attention deficit hyperactivity disorder or A.D.H.D.	~	a condition involving inattention, difficulty focusing to complete tasks as well as organizing projects, fidgeting, distractability, forgetfulness, verbal impulsivity, intrusiveness, and/ or excessive movements
autism	(aw-tizm)	social interaction impairment that includes lack of peer relationships, spontaneous sharing, and/ or social reciprocation
bipolar	(bi-po-lar)	a potentially psychotic genetic disorder characterized by recurrent major depressive and manic episodes that present pronounced mood fluctuations
cataplexy	(cat-a-plex-e)	the process of sudden loss of all muscle tone, especially when experiencing intense emotions
catatonic	(kat-a-ton-ik)	related to motor immobility
compliance	(kom-pli-ans)	willingness to go along with recommended treatment, etc.
cyclothymia	(si-klo-thi-me-a)	related to a chronic, fluctuating mood disorder involving hypomanic and mild depressive symptoms
dementia	(de-men-che-a)	multiple cognitive deficits that result in significant impairment in functioning
dysmorphic	(dis-mor-fik)	related to excessive distress and painful preoccupation with an imagined defect in appearance
dyspareunia	(dis-par-ew-ne-a)	related to recurrent difficult or painful male/female sexual intercourse
dysthymia	(dis-thi-me-a)	related to chronically difficult and depressed daily mood for at least two years involving changes in sleep and appetite, poor focus, fatigue and hopelessness
echolalia	(e-ko-la-le-a)	related to repetition of anything verbalized
echopraxia	(e-ko-prax-e-a)	related to involuntary imitation of another's movement

TERMS	PRONOUNCIATIONS	DEFINITIONS
encopresis	(en-ko-pre-sis)	inappropriate and repetitive uncontrolled fecal passage
enuresis	(en-yur-e-sis)	involuntary or intentional urination on clothes or bed wetting after age 7 years
exhibitionism	(x-hi-bi-shun-izm)	related to persistent, intense sexual arousal with fantasies, urges, and behaviors related to exposing one's genitals to a stranger
frotteurism	(frot-er-izm)	recurrent, intense sexual arousal involving urges, fantasies, and/or actions of touching as well rubbing against a non-consentual person
histrionic	(his-tri-on-ik)	related to uncomfortable feeling if no the center of attention, exaggerated expressions, and tending toward bein provocative or sexually seductive
hypersomnia	(hi-per-som-ne-a)	related to excessive sleep episodes fo a month minimum
insomnia	(in-som-ne-a)	related to difficulty initiating or maintaining a restorative sleep for at least a one month period
masochism	(mas-o-kizm)	sexual arousal via urges, fantasies, or real actions of being belittled, humiliated, tied and/or beaten
megalomania	(meg-al-o-ma-ne-a)	related to delusion of overevaluation of self (for example; as king, God or president)
narcissistic	(nar-sis-is-tik)	a tendency toward an entitlement sensibility requiring much admiration arrogance, exploitative of others, and lacking empathy
narcolepsy	(nar-ko-lep-se)	chronic process involving involuntary episodes of sleeping (with REM)
neurotic	(ner-ot-ik)	related to nerves and associated potential emotional issues
obsessive compulsive disorder or O.C.D.	(ob-ses-iv kom-pul-siv)	a disorder in which anxiety producing thoughts, impulses, or images are denied, suppressed, or neutralized wit other thoughts or repetitive behaviors aimed at returning to being less anxious
pandiculation	(pan-dik-u-la-shun)	stretching and yawning
pedophilia	(ped-o-fil-e-a)	related to recurrent, strong sexual arousal involving urges, fantasies and behaviors of sexual activity with a prepubescent child (five years or older)

TERMS	PRONOUNCIATIONS	DEFINITIONS
phobia	(fo-be-a)	related to a persistent, excessive, and/ or unreasonable fear that interferes with daily functioning and is fueled by the anticipation of a specific event or object
agoraphobia	(a-gor-a-fo-be-a)	an irrational fear involving difficulty leaving home or a familiar setting
ailurophobia	(al-ur-o-fo-be-a)	an irrational fear of cats
anthophobia	(an-tho-fo-be-a)	an irrational fear of flowers
arachnophobia	(a-rak-no-fo-be-a)	an irrational fear of spiders
aviophobia	(av-i-o-fo-be-a)	an irrational fear of flying
catagelophobia	(cat-a-gel-o-fo-be-a)	an irrational fear of being ridiculed
chirophobia	(ki-ro-fo-be-a)	an irrational fear of shaking hands
euphobia	(ew-fo-be-a)	an irrational fear of good news
mysophobia	(mis-o-fo-be-a)	an irrational fear of germs
psychotic	(si-kot-ik)	related to the condition of impaired ego boundaries and severe distortion/ impairment to reality testing
post traumatic stress disorder or P.T.S.D.	(post-traw-mat-ik stress)	a disorder involving persistent involuntary re-experiencing of a traumatic event, emotional numbness, hypervigilance, insomnia, difficulty concentrating, social estrangement, increased startle reflex, and limited affect
adism	(sa-dizm)	related to sexual arousal via urges, fantasies, or real actions involving physical or psychological suffering
eparation anxiety	(sep-ar-a-shun)	excessive anxiety concerning separation from home and/ or attachment figure
chizophrenia	(skiz-o-fren-e-a)	related to a psychotic disorder involving delusions, hallucinations, social withdrawal and disorganized speech/behavior
ic	(tik)	a recurrent, rapid, and sudden motor movement or vocalization
ourette's syndrome	(tur-etz)	a disorder characterized by involuntary motor and/or vocal tics that do not relent for three consecutive months, compromise functioning and cause remarkable distress
ansvestic fetishism	(trans-ves-tik)	related to recurrent sexual arousal of a heterosexual male involving cross dressing
agismus	(va-jin-is-mus)	related to a recurrent involuntary muscular spasm in the outside third of the vagina that impairs sexual intercourse

TERMS	PRONOUNCIATIONS	DEFINITIONS
voyeurism	(voy-ur-izm)	related to sexual arousal involving the act of observing another person nude, becoming undressed, or engaging in a sexual act

GENERAL EATING DISORDERS		
anorexia nervosa	(an-or-ex-e-a ner-vo-sa)	an eating disorder characterized by a distorted body image, compulsive control, food aversion, fear of weight gain, and layering of clothing (higher death rate than other psychiatric eating issues)
binge eating disorder	(bing e-ting)	eating in excess of 2500 calories within 2 hours with feelings of shame, distress, and physical discomfort at least biweekly for 6 months (beyond hunger, eating to cope with stress)
bulimia nervosa	(bul-e-me-a ner-vo-sa)	an eating disorder involving chronic secretive uncontrolled bingeing during brief amount of time followed by self induced purging with substance abuse, gag reflex stimulation, and/or intense exercise for at least 2 weeks over a 3 week period
diabulimia	(di-a-bul-e-me-a)	deliberate decreased insulin dose given by Type 1 diabetics to themselves for the purpose of losing weight

ABBREVIATIONS	DEFINITIONS
AD	Alzheimer's disease
ADD	Attention Deficit Disorder
ADHD	Attention Deficit Hyperactivity Disorder
ALS	amyotrophic lateral sclerosis or Lou Gehrig's disease
BD	brain dead
BEAM	brain electrical activity mapping
CJD	Creutzfeldt-Jakob or Mad Cow disease
CNS	central nervous system
CP	cerebral palsy
CSF	cerebrospinal fluid
DT	delirium tremors
ECT	electroconvulsive therapy
EEG	electroencephalogram
EST	electric shock therapy
GAD	generalized anxiety disorder
HD	Huntington's disease
LOC	loss of consciousness
LP	lumbar puncture or spinal tap
MBD	minimal brain dysfunction
MS	multiple sclerosis
NTD	neural tube defect
OBS	organic brain syndrome
OCD	obsessive compulsive disorder
PD	Parkinson's disease

ABBREVIATIONS	DEFINITIONS
’NS	peripheral nervous system
’TSD	post traumatic stress disorder
;AD	seasonal affective disorder
;Z	seizure
'BI	traumatic brain injury
'ENS	transcutaneous electrical nerve stimulation
'IA	transient ischemic attack

’RACTICE, PRACTICE, PRACTICE...........

:xercise 1:

s soon as you have received new medical terms, begin to review. Using blank 3”X5” index cards, create flashcards to view all of the new medical terms in this chapter by writing each of the correctly spelled terms five times on one side of e index card and the definition of each term on the other side of the index card. Keeping all of these cards in your right ›cket, continually review all of the cards throughout the day. Whenever you have learned a card, place it in your left ›cket. After you have learned all of these new terms, periodically refresh your memory with review.

:xercise 2:

:rbal Portrait. Write a one paragraph synopsis of what behavior one would imagine witnessing when observing each of ve differently diagnosed psychiatric patients (for a total of five paragraphs).

:xercise 3:

› Comply or Not. In a one page paper, explain the issues of medication compliance for a fifty-five year old bipolar tient with a history of C.H.F. and T.I.A. who is now exhibiting early sx of dementia.

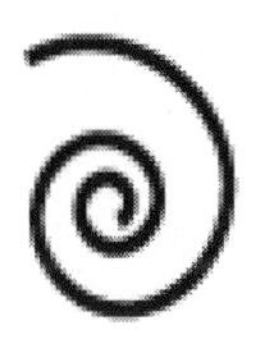